MEN'S PRIVATE PARTS

*A Pocket Reference to Prostate,
Urologic, and Sexual Health*

James H. Gilbaugh, Jr., M.D.

A FIRESIDE BOOK

Published by Simon & Schuster

New York London Toronto Sydney Singapore

FIRESIDE
Rockefeller Center
1230 Avenue of the Americas
New York, NY 10020

For information about special discounts for bulk purchases,
please contact Simon & Schuster Special Sales:
1-800-456-6798 or business@simonandschuster.com

Designed by Lauren Simonetti

Manufactured in the United States of America

1   3   5   7   9   10   8   6   4   2

Library of Congress Cataloging-in-Publication Data
Gilbaugh, James H.
Men's private parts : a pocket reference to prostate, urologic, and sexual health /
James H. Gilbaugh, Jr.
p.   cm.
Includes index.
1. Andrology—Popular works.   2. Generative organs, Male—Popular works.
3. Men—Health and hygiene—Popular works.   I. Title.
RC881 .G539   2002
616.6'5—dc21   2002017674

ISBN 0-7432-1344-0

An earlier edition of this book was published as *A Doctor's Guide to Men's Private Parts*.

*This book is dedicated to my wife, Marilyn,
and to my family, as well as to my teachers and patients.*

CONTENTS

INTRODUCTION

The same questions asked over and over by my patients led me to search for a book to help satisfy their curiosity. I found nothing in print that filled the bill, and this led to the creation of this book, which describes the private parts of the male body and how those parts function. It details how they work separately and together, how they can go haywire, and whether they can be repaired or replaced. And to make the book accessible, I wrote it in basic, everyday, real-people language.

You have been urinating since birth and thinking nothing of it; it comes naturally. As you mature, you don't have to know anything about sex to experience it, for it too is one of nature's urges. For most men, the dual yet separate function of the penis is performed for years without problems. Still, the aging process begins at birth, and as we grow older, parts weaken and malfunction: an erection fades or it doesn't happen at all; urine flow is restricted or blocked; blood appears in the semen or urine. Obviously, something is wrong when any of these things happen. It's in such instances that an idea about what may be happening and what you can do about it is reassuring.

The drawing below identifies and locates the male anatomy, internal and external. The penis and the testicles are fa-

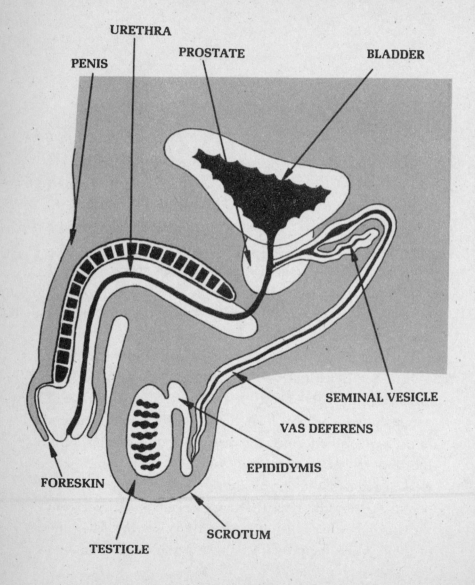

miliar, but the third organ, the prostate gland, is less so. All operate automatically when the brain sends down its signal. This efficient system ordinarily works well for years, but as men age the prostate gland may become enlarged, the penis may fail to become erect, and the testicles may develop any number of problems. Fortunately, most malfunctions can be repaired. Prostate obstruction can be relieved, artificial erections can be created, and most testicle problems can be treated; more in-depth discussions of problems and their solutions are contained here.

In summary, *Men's Private Parts* describes the function of men's private parts and accessories. Through its guidance, you will be able to recognize and anticipate potential problems and know when to seek appropriate repairs. In addition, trouble spots will be identified and solutions will be presented.

Finally, along with this information and advice come the experiences of real men and some self-inventory.

Chapter 10 presents the results of a lifestyle survey reporting the sexual expectations and experiences of a group of men aged thirty-five to fifty years. Men should try the quizzes in Chapter 12 and compare results with the men I surveyed. Ladies who are interested in learning how men operate may be surprised to read the results and comparisons.

The pages ahead are packed with clear, useful information. Men and women alike are invited to read on and make those private parts become familiar parts.

Men's
Private
Parts

CHAPTER ONE

TROUBLESHOOTING

Problem 1: My penis isn't big enough.
Answer: No man thinks his penis is big enough. Penis size, however, has nothing to do with climax or orgasm. (See chapter 3.)

Problem 2: I take longer to realize an erection now than I did when I was younger.
Answer: Possibly. Erections are reached most quickly during adolescence, the years of spontaneous erections. As a man ages beyond his thirties or forties, direct stimulation of the penis may be required to produce an erection. (See chapter 3.)

Problem 3: My erections are not as stiff as they were when I was younger.
Answer: This is often true. The firmest erections are reached during adolescence; hormones and blood vessels operate differently after teen years have passed. A certain reduction in stiffness may be expected. (See chapter 3.)

Problem 4: I can't get one erection after another, as I once could.

Answer: The refractory period, the time it takes to get another erection after ejaculation and orgasm, increases with age. It is very brief for a teenager, but can be twenty-four hours in later years. This is normal. (See chapter 2.)

Problem 5: I lose my erection during sex more frequently than before.

Answer: Again, this may be a result of the aging process at work. Lack of concentration, distracting noises, fear of interruption, and other environmental influences—including your partner—can affect performance. (See chapter 5.)

Problem 6: My penis requires more stimulation than in the past to reach orgasm.

Answer: Through the aging process, again, all things slow down. This includes sensitivity, nerve conduction, and blood-vessel activity. As a man ages, more stimulation is needed for orgasm. (See chapter 3.)

Problem 7: I will become impotent if I have a prostate operation.

Answer: Not true. Most prostate operations should not interrupt a man's ability to have an erection and successful intercourse. (See chapters 2 and 7.)

Problem 8: Prostate operations are painful.

Answer: Not true. Most men fear this operation because they think it is very painful, but it isn't. The operation is usually performed under a spinal anesthetic, which allows complete consciousness without pain. (See chapter 7.)

Problem 9: Isolated periods of impotence indicate impending doom.

Answer: Not true. Isolated episodes of impotence can happen during sexual encounters at any age and are not unusual. These blank periods usually are associated with stressful situations, initial sexual encounters, or alcohol or drug overuse. (See chapter 5.)

Problem 10: I am done if I fail to reach orgasm.

Answer: Not so. As a man ages, it is not uncommon to fail to reach orgasm during sex at least occasionally. But it is also easier to get another erection if there was no ejaculation with the last one. (See chapter 2.)

Problem 11: I ejaculate a smaller amount of semen than I once did.

Answer: True. A decrease in volume of ejaculate is normal as a man ages. Older men, in their seventies and eighties, may not ejaculate at all but still have orgasms. (See chapter 2.)

Problem 12: Ejaculation is not effective unless it is powerful.

Answer: Not true. In a man's prime, ejaculate can spurt two feet, but the process loses vigor as age affects muscle and nerve functions and blood supplies. (See chapter 2.)

Problem 13: I'm afraid that masturbation when I was younger, or even now, may affect my sexual functioning in the future.

Answer: Nonsense. Lack of education and feelings of guilt promote myths of this sort, which have no basis in scientific fact. (See chapter 2.)

Problem 14: Alcohol inhibits my sexual ability.

Answer: Maybe. Alcohol in small amounts can stimulate interest in sex, but in larger amounts it is a depressant and can cause impaired function and even impotence. (See chapter 5.)

Problem 15: As I get older, my penis gets smaller.

Answer: Untrue. As you get older, your stomach gets fatter, so proportionately your penis looks smaller. No kidding; it's an optical illusion. (See chapter 3.)

Problem 16: If I have serious heart trouble—a heart attack or cardiac-bypass surgery—my sex life will be over.

Answer: Not so. It is not necessary to forgo sexual activity after a heart attack; most men can resume sex without any serious effects after such events. (See chapter 5.)

Problem 17: Masturbation makes me feel guilty.

Answer: Masturbation is an important part of a person's sexuality. Men and women, married and single, young and old, do it. (See chapter 2.)

Problem 18: Will smoking reduce my sexual ability?

Answer: Yes. Nicotine can constrict small blood vessels and has a dampening effect on a man's erectile ability immediate as well as long term. (See chapter 5.)

Problem 19: Recreational drugs get me in the mood for sex, but they are dangerous.

Answer: Marijuana, cocaine, ecstasy, and amphetamines can increase sexual desire and lower inhibitions in the short run, but over time can cause impotence and other serious hazards to health. (See chapter 5.)

Problem 20: I have arthritis. Will sex help?
Answer: It might. Many patients find relief for four to six hours after having an orgasm. (See chapter 2.)

Problem 21: My ulcer medication makes me impotent.
Answer: This is a common complaint among patients being treated for ulcers with certain drugs that have the side effect of blocking male hormone production. (See chapter 5.)

Problem 22: Blood pressure pills make me impotent.
Answer: Possibly. Medicines used to treat high blood pressure limit pressure required for an erection, so difficulties may result. (See chapter 5.)

Problem 23: Is a person who tests negative for AIDS a safe sex partner?
Answer: Absolutely not. A negative test for HIV antibody is no guarantee that an individual cannot transmit AIDS. There is a lag time of six months or longer after infection occurs before the blood test shows positive. Safe-sex clubs won't prevent AIDS. (See chapter 8.)

Problem 24: Can an oral pill help impotence or erectile dysfunction?
Answer: Yes. Viagra (sildenafil citrate) has now been approved by the FDA for use in treating male impotence. (See chapter 5.)

Problem 25: A vasectomy will cause hardening of the arteries, heart disease, or other diseases.

Answer: Not true. A study of 10,000 sterilized men conducted by the National Institutes of Health found no increased risk of developing any such disorders among the participants. (See chapter 2.)

Problem 26: If I have prostate obstruction, I'm going to need prostate surgery.
Answer: Not true. Many medical and nonsurgical techniques developed in recent years may allow a man to avoid prostate surgery. (See chapter 7.)

Problem 27: Sex before athletic competition will wreck me!
Answer: Not true. (See chapter 2.)

Problem 28: My urinary flow has decreased and it seems like I have to get up at night more to urinate. Is all of this part of just getting older?
Answer: Possibly. See chapter 12 and take the results of the two tests to your physician. (See chapter 12.)

CHAPTER TWO

EJACULATION, CONDOMS, AND VASECTOMY

On reaching puberty, a boy soon discovers that he can get an erection and that, with a little stroking, his erection can produce ejaculate and a new feeling called orgasm. The erection is commonly called, among other names, a hard-on, and the sticky fluid that spurts out is called come or cum.

Masturbation is usually the earliest form of adolescent experimentation with the mysteries of sex. It also is probably the scariest, owing to the vacuum of ignorance that affiliates it with temptation and evil. No, it won't make you crazy or affect your adult sex life: masturbation is the shock absorber of puberty, easing the bumps of adolescent development.

A boy's penis will become erect while he's asleep during the night. This is a nocturnal erection, a normal, automatic function. Frequently, this erection will produce a nocturnal emission, called a wet dream. That's okay, too. The wet dream relieves pressure in a male body that produces semen but has no place for it to go.

Maria, a nurse on our hospital day shift, raised five boys through their teens. She once talked to me about their different reactions to nocturnal emissions, from boy to boy and time to time. All seemed to fear discovery of their bedding after a wet dream; one had gone so far as to wash his own sheets before his mother got up in the morning, trying to keep his starchy secret from her.

I assured her that nocturnal emissions were healthy indications of manhood and told her that she ought to reassure her sons. She said later that she'd had a good conversation with them, explaining some of the ways a boy naturally becomes a man and thereby putting an end to any guilt—and midnight laundry activity.

Not only teens but most males, in fact, have erections regularly through the night. This occurs from infancy through old age, so long as a man is capable of erection. A normal, healthy man will have about five erections during a night's sleep, spaced an hour to an hour and a half apart and lasting twenty to thirty minutes each. Usually, the only evidence of all this activity is the erection a man finds when he awakens in the morning and feels a need to urinate. His bladder erection, or "piss hard-on," is actually his last erectile achievement of the night. Nocturnal erections are more prevalent and of longer duration during youth, but as years pass, they become shorter and fewer in number.

For a man doubting his erectile function, a test of whether or not he can still get an erection is to learn what happens at night. A simple but effective method of doing so is to stick perforated but unseparated postage stamps around the limp penis at bedtime and see in the morning if the stamps have been separated by an erection. A more elaborate snap gauge is available commercially, but stamps will do just as well.

Scientists have identified two kinds of sleep: dreaming sleep and nondreaming sleep. These alternate during the night; most men experience both kinds. Dreaming sleep is also called REM (for rapid eye movement) sleep, because eyes move rapidly and seem almost to jump during these phases. Most erections occur during REM sleep.

The amount of fluid men ejaculate and the force at which they do it decrease with age. Eventually, ejaculate may barely reach beyond the penis. But there are aberrations. In some cases, ejaculate doesn't come until after intercourse or masturbation is completed; in other cases, it doesn't come at all. The volume of fluid in each ejaculation can vary from 1.5 to 5.0 cubic centimeters, with the average being 3.0 cc, or about a teaspoonful. (With age, volume peters out and sometimes even disappears altogether.) The ejaculate squirts out in several whitish, jellylike clumps. Very rapidly after exiting the body, the gel is liquefied by an enzyme to an opaque watery fluid. This liquid form aids the sperm on its trip to the female egg for fertilization.

One of nature's anomalies is the wide variation of ejaculate volume produced among animals. A bull elephant, for example, produces a prodigious amount, as might be expected: he's good for more than 300 cc, or more than a cup. A stallion produces 70 cc. A man's production is well below the average production of a dog, which is 20 cc.

Contrary to common belief, the testicles are not the major source of ejaculate. Seminal vesicles, small pouches behind the bladder and the prostate, produce about two-thirds of ejaculate volume; about one-third is produced by the prostate. Less than one percent is produced by the testicles, which do produce all sperm. Yet despite their small proportional contribution to ejaculate volume, the sperm cells produced in the testicles number from 40 million to 200 million per cubic centimeter of fluid, translating into 120 million to 600 million cells in each ejaculation.

Among other minor contributors are Cowper's glands, paired pea-size glands directly below the prostate, which drain into the urethral tube. These were first identified by William Cowper in 1698. After almost three centuries, medical science still does not fully understand their function. (One fact about Cowper's glands is certain, however: they produce drops of seminal fluid that appear at the head of the penis during sexual arousal but before ejaculation. These secretions often contain live sperm, so they make risky any birth-control plan that depends on withdrawal before ejaculation.)

EJACULATORY CONTROL

Normal ejaculation occurs simultaneously with orgasm. There are three principal forms of abnormal ejaculation: premature, retarded, and retrograde.

Coming too soon may be the least troublesome of these aberrations, but it is perhaps the most frustrating. Consider the guy who made a visit to a prostitute and came in a basin while she was washing his penis, or the man who climaxes before his partner has even become aroused—serious problems can result. The remedy for premature ejaculation usually comes with practiced patience, assisted by counseling if the problem persists. Sex counselors Masters and Johnson have suggested a squeeze technique to remedy the situation, saying that a momentary squeeze of the penis just before ejaculation becomes inevitable conditions a man's response and delays or postpones his ejaculation.

The opposite problem, retarded ejaculation, happens less often. It is seen particularly among older men. Psychological problems may result, but a more typical effect is that a couple simply gets tired from having to work longer and harder.

Retrograde ejaculation differs from the other forms because it has nothing to do with timing and its effect is permanent. It happens when the opening from the bladder does not close during erection and semen spurts backward into the bladder. The wrong-way semen later is passed with urination. To ascertain ejaculation, urine is sampled after ejaculation for sperm count.

Retrograde ejaculation frequently follows a prostatectomy, but it can also result from injuries to nerves following bowel, pelvic, or colon surgery. Retrograde ejaculation may also be caused by diabetes—indeed, backward ejaculation may be an early sign of diabetes—or nerve diseases. A man experiencing retrograde ejaculation can still climax and feel the effects, but a woman can't be fertilized. Certain medications can reverse the problem temporarily.

Victor, aged seventy and a little on the stubborn side, had been sexually active prior to his prostate operation. He came in for his six-week postoperative prostate checkup with the news that he could get erections but couldn't ejaculate. His only problem, as it turned out, was that he hadn't read the instruction sheet he got when he was discharged from the hospital.

The sheet explained that he could expect normal intercourse and normal orgasm, but no ejaculation. Victor's wife volunteered that she had read the postop material and knew all about his retrograde ejaculation. He was just one of those guys who wanted assurance from his doctor that everything was as it should be. I've heard from some couples that they prefer this reverse effect, as it isn't so messy.

SEX AND ATHLETIC PERFORMANCE

The myth that sex shortly before a big event will hurt, even wreck, an athlete's performance has been handed down for generations. The theory was that abstinence leads to frustration, which produces aggression, causing more vigor on the playing field. To my knowledge, there is no scientific study of athletes that shows this to be true. As a urologist who has among his patients both amateur and professional athletes, I know of no athlete who felt he or she needed to avoid sex before competition. In fact, it is fairly well accepted that sex the night before an athletic event, if anything, is beneficial for the athlete—It's the best natural sleeping pill! I subscribe to the theory that sex doesn't wreck you, attributed to Alexander the Great and expressed well by Bill Bowerman, a former United States Olympic track and field coach: It's not the getting it that kills you, it's the chasing after it!

INFERTILITY

Infertility, the inability to reproduce, is more common than generally believed, occurring for example, in 10 to 15 percent of marriages. A couple may be considered infertile if no pregnancy occurs after a year or two of unprotected intercourse, or intercourse without use of contraception. The husband, if he proves to be the source of the problem, may find that he is shooting blanks for one of several possible reasons, among them an ineffective sperm count, a complete absence of live sperm, or retrograde ejaculation.

ARTIFICIAL INSEMINATION

For a select group of patients, artificial insemination may be the best way to induce pregnancy, as sperm that bypass the vagina may have better success in swimming up the fallopian tube and impregnating the female egg.

Electrically stimulated ejaculation, a technique developed for use on animals, is now being applied successfully to humans. A probe in the rectum can stimulate ejaculation, even in cases of spinal-cord injuries where normal ejaculation would be impossible.

PAIN RELIEVER?

Some patients report that orgasm can relieve their arthritic pain for one to six hours. This may be because hormone releases during orgasm produce something like runner's high, or it may be that orgasm blocks pain receptors in the brain with a cortisone-like substance.

ABSTINENCE

Long-term abstinence or nonuse of erections can create anxiety, but normal physical functioning should return to the male if all systems—vascular, neurovascular, and hormonal—are intact. However, postmenopausal women who have not had intercourse for an extended time are likely to be affected by vaginal atrophy and constriction. Various treatments are available, but the most effective is a cooperative and patient partner.

CONDOMS

More than $200 million worth of condoms are sold in the United States each year, perhaps one-third of them to women. Condoms' current popularity results from their proven efficiency in preventing sexually transmitted diseases (STDs).

Though condoms' effectiveness in blocking common STDs was well known, the alarming epidemic of AIDS (acquired immunodeficiency syndrome) stimulated interest in and widespread use of condoms over the past couple of decades because condoms offer almost assured protection from the human immunodeficiency virus (HIV), which causes AIDS. This virus is carried by body fluids (blood, semen, and vaginal secretions) that leave one partner and enter vulnerable openings (vagina, rectum, urethra) of the other. Condoms act as a barrier to transmission of body fluids.

Tips on Condom Use

- Don't use an old condom. Condoms should have an expiration date stamped on the package; they have a safe shelf life of two years. Don't stretch your luck.
- Condoms are highly effective in blocking sexually transmitted diseases, but they are not foolproof. Remember, an uncovered herpes sore—such as one not on but near the penis—can escape a condom's coverage.
- Proper and consistent use of condoms is 90 percent effective in preventing pregnancy.
- Proper and consistent use of condoms is required for prevention of sexually transmitted diseases.
- To use a condom effectively:
  - Place the correct side of the condom against the head of the penis. You'll know you have the wrong side if the condom won't unroll.
  - Unroll the condom over an erect penis from head to base; allow a one-half-inch space at the closed (head) end if there is no reservoir.
  - Put on the condom prior to foreplay, before the penis touches the vagina, mouth, or rectum.
  - After ejaculation, remove the condom before the erection wilts; avoid spilling contents.
- Use only a water-based lubricant (such as K-Y jelly) with a condom; a petroleum-based lubricant, such as Vaseline, may damage latex material.
- Never use a condom more than once.
- Keep condoms cool; do not store them in a wallet or glove compartment.
- Don't be bashful about buying condoms.
- Don't fill condoms with water and drop them from hotel-room windows.

The AIDS-induced revival of condoms, which had fallen from favor with the development of birth-control pills, has in effect given condoms a second purpose. Although condom packages once had a label reading SOLD FOR THE PREVENTION OF DISEASE ONLY, they were bought—in drugstores, barbershops, and men's-room vending machines—primarily by men who wanted sex but not pregnant girlfriends. Now, once again, they are bought and sold explicitly for disease protection as well as birth control. Used properly and consistently,

How to Use a Condom

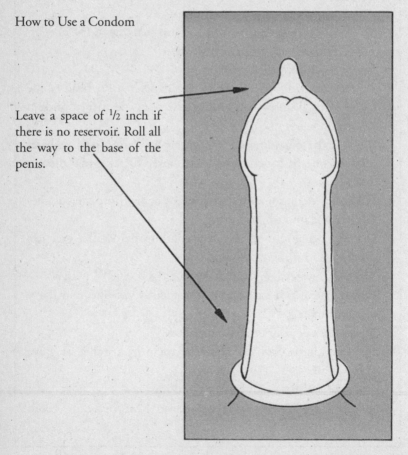

Leave a space of ½ inch if there is no reservoir. Roll all the way to the base of the penis.

condoms are 90 percent effective in preventing both pregnancy and sexually transmitted diseases.

A condom is a latex-rubber sheath that rolls tightly over an erect penis. Also called a prophylactic or skin, it is a modern version of a lambskin cecum (pouch) believed by many to have been invented in England in the eighteenth century by a Dr. Condom—who may or may not have actually existed.

Some condoms still are made from membranes of animal intestines. These are especially comfortable, but their natural pores cannot assure protection against virus or bacteria penetration. Other condom materials have been introduced, but most have been manufactured from latex rubber since that process was introduced in the 1930s.

More than one hundred brands of condoms are made and sold in the United States. Most are seven or eight inches long and are rolled and packaged individually in plastic or foil. There are two principal designs: some have reservoir ends to hold ejaculate and some do not; some are coated with lubricant and some are not.

Condoms are also sold in assorted colors, some even in assorted flavors. They are available with "French tickler" and other accessories, and with plain or ribbed sides, supposedly to provide varying degrees of sensitivity. Condoms may even be purchased with an adhesive ring that fits around the base of the penis to prevent the condom from slipping off if the erection subsides.

Condoms manufactured in the United States must meet federal specifications for material and labeling. The shelf life of a condom is two years; an expiration date should be stamped on the package.

VASECTOMY

Medical science has developed two more emission-control techniques: vasectomy and the sperm-bank deposit.

Vasectomy is a simple, safe, and effective birth-control method that blocks the flow of sperm into the seminal fluid by surgically cutting the tube, or vas deferens—which carries sperm from the testes to the urethra—in the scrotum. The operation is most often conducted in a doctor's office, requires only a local anesthetic, and can be completed in fifteen or twenty minutes. Pain usually is minimal and discomfort disappears after a day or two.

The operation is totally effective in almost all cases, but some time is required to clear sperm already in the body's distribution system before the operation. For this reason, the patient must return for sperm counts until an examination of semen, obtained by masturbation, shows that the sperm count is zero. Usually a first check is made one month after the operation and another is made in two months. Today, vasectomies are performed on more than a half million men in the United States every year. It is safer than the more complicated tubal ligation, the comparable operation on a woman.

After vasectomy, your manliness will not be affected. There is no effect on levels of testosterone, the male hormone produced by the testes; your sexual functioning will not be altered. Your ability to have an erection and orgasm will not be changed, nor will the amount of semen ejaculated be noticeably decreased. In fact, some patients say their sexual functioning is improved after vasectomy because the fear of unwanted pregnancy is relieved.

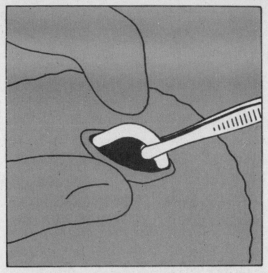

Vas deferens is identified through scrotal incision.

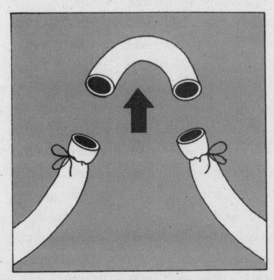

Both ends of the vas deferens are tied; at the option of the physician, the segment may or may not be removed.

Articles suggesting a relationship between vasectomy and prostate cancer have appeared both in the lay press and in medical literature over the last decade. Reports have also incriminated vasectomy as the cause of an increased risk of heart disease. Subsequent publications, however, have refuted these links and the National Institute of Health has recommended no change in vasectomy practice.

Vasectomy should be considered a long-term, permanent method of male contraception. Hence, before a vasectomy is performed, it is critical that the patient determine that he wishes to father no more children, as the operation is intended to be irreversible. The patient should consider the possibilities of divorce and remarriage, however improbable they might seem to be. And after such consideration, the operation must be authorized by the patient and endorsed by his wife, in both cases by written statements.

No scalpel vasectomies have been performed in China for years, now in the United States for the last several years. The technique involves performing a vasectomy through a single puncture wound, and the result is the same as the vasectomy done in the usual manner. The vas deferens is cut as in the standard vasectomy already described.

Again, a vasectomy is generally meant to be forever, but recently reversals of vasectomy have been performed with some success. An operation to rejoin the vas deferens tubes, called a vasovasostomy or reanastomosis has attracted the interest of men who have changed their minds. This operation is more complex and more expensive than the original vasectomy, and results are mixed. A high percentage of men who have had the operation have delivered sperm, but the pregnancy rate is variable, apparently depending greatly on the expertise and experience of the urologist performing the surgery and the fertility of the woman. Evidence indicates that this highly technical surgery is more likely to be successful if performed by a specially trained urologist rather than a nonspecialist.

Another way to hedge one's bets in the face of the permanency of a vasectomy is to store sperm before the operation. Frozen-sperm banks are becoming more popular, but their success in inducing pregnancy remains to be seen.

INFERTILITY

Fertility problems in men are related to the production, quality, and movement of sperm. Any number of factors can influence male infertility; among the most common are the following:

- *Caffeine:* Caffeine, found in coffee as well as in many soft drinks and medications, appears to make sperm sluggish and slow.
- *Alcohol:* Too much alcohol lowers production of testosterone, a critical male sex hormone.
- *Smoking:* Tobacco smoke lowers sperm count and slows sperm motility.
- *Drugs:* Recreational drugs, including marijuana, may decrease testosterone levels.
- *Jeans, shorts, and underwear:* Tight jeans or shorts can overheat sperm-producing cells in testicles, lowering sperm count.
- *Hot tubs:* Frequent tub use can lower sperm count by overheating sperm-producing cells.

- *Age:* Sperm production drops sharply after age thirty—but can persist at lower levels into the nineties.
- *Cimetidine:* This drug, prescribed for treatment of ulcers, also decreases testosterone level.
- *Diethylstilbestrol:* This drug, used thirty to forty years ago to prevent miscarriages, was later found to cause fertility problems among men born to mothers who used it.
- *Vaginal douches:* Douches, sprays, and lubricants containing certain chemicals can immobilize sperm.
- *STDs and Infection:* All sexually transmitted diseases can affect fertility adversely, as can other infections.
- *Diabetes:* Nerve and vascular damage caused by diabetes can induce retrograde ejaculation, in which sperm is not delivered.

CHAPTER THREE

THE PENIS

The penis is a complex organ, particularly when it comes to its erectile capacity. Blood pumped from all over the body contributes to an erection, or hard-on, in three steps. First, nerve stimuli cause the muscles in the walls of tiny penile blood vessels to relax and thus accommodate greater blood volume in the organ. Then, the penis gains erectness and stiffness as three tubes that run its length engorge with blood. Two of these tubes, spongy tissue called corpora cavernosa, absorb most of the blood, while some goes to a third tube, the corpus spongiosum, which is the covering of the urethra, itself the tube that runs through the penis and carries semen and urine. Once filled, the penis traps the blood inside to maintain the erection. Blood volume in an erection is six to eight times the normal flow to the penis. Any malfunction of the nerves, blood vessels, or other tissues serving the penis can cause an erectile problem.

The product of this process is, of course, an erection, the size of which is the most frequently expressed concern of men regarding their penises. Male erections generally range from four and a half inches to eight inches, but most are six inches, and most men wish their erections were bigger. But that aside, other concerns include minor bends in the erect penis, technically called chordee, which are not uncommon. These do not interfere with function, though surgery may be necessary to correct severe chordee.

Some helpful statistics about erections were amassed by an enterprising lady who worked in a massage parlor. She put the tape to the erections of 1,681 of her customers, presumably as part of her warm-up routine, and published her findings in *Playboy*. Her research indicated that 97 percent of the men she measured achieved erections of the average six inches; only seven came up to eight inches. Still, a fact that many if not most men are reluctant to accept is that penis size is for the most part irrelevant to sexual satisfaction for either a male or female. Nature placed the sensitive nerve endings that facilitate orgasm at the most practical point possible— up front: on a man they are at the head (glans) of his penis; on a woman they are at a protrusion above the opening of the vagina (clitoris). Stimulation, not depth of thrust, is all that is needed.

Alex, a fifty-four-year-old photographer, confided that he had always been embarrassed because he thought his penis was too small. Even with a full erection he couldn't get a condom to stay on unless he first wrapped a Kleenex around his penis. I assured him that no matter what its size, his penis was big enough to have intercourse. Hundreds of times, I've heard a man complain about his penis size—but never because it was too big.

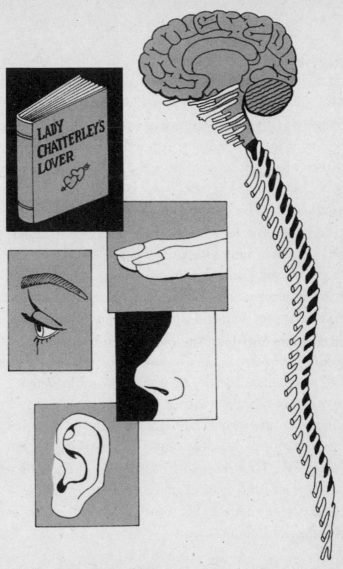

The making of an erection—the brain is probably the largest sex organ in man. Many elements, including psyche, touch, sight, smell, and hearing, are important for initiating and maintaining an erection. Some think that smell is the most important, but this is debatable.

CIRCUMCISION

Usually performed shortly after birth, circumcision is the surgical removal of the foreskin that covers the head of the penis. The practice dates back to 4000 B.C. among tribal cultures in several parts of the world. Today, it is performed for religious or medical reasons. Among Jews, for instance, circumcision has long and still symbolizes Abraham's covenant with God, as stated in the Book of Genesis: "Every male among you shall be circumcised. You shall be circumcised in the flesh of your foreskins, and it shall be a sign of the covenant between me and you" (Gen. 17:10–11).

In the United States, circumcision is a fairly routine procedure for nonreligious as well as religious reasons. The custom is much less prevalent in Europe, although a few operations are performed based on medical opinion. And while medical opinion is in fact undecided about the use of circumcision for health reasons and debate on the relationship between circumcision and cancer a source of diverse opinions and conflicting scientific proofs, the fact nevertheless remains that the great majority of penile cancer victims were not circumcised at birth. Thus it seems reasonable to suggest circumcision as a precaution against such a devastating disease.

Be that as it may, there is some agreement on medical issues concerning circumcision:

- There is no proof that circumcision protects against venereal disease.
- There is conflicting evidence regarding cancer of the cervix in sexual partners of uncircumcised men.

- Circumcision may prevent penile cancer, though proper retraction of foreskin and cleansing of the penis also appears to be a means of prevention.
- In young boys, those who are not circumcised show a significant increase in urinary-tract infections when compared to rates for circumcised boys.
- Meatitis (inflammation of the opening of the urethra) and meatal stenosis occur more frequently in circumcised boys than they do in uncircumcised boys.
- Injuries from circumcision are rare but do occur and vary greatly in severity. Occasionally such injury will require an additional procedure to be corrected.

Circumcision is a simple excision of the foreskin. Infection, should it occur, can easily be treated with an antibiotic ointment. Significant injury to the penis itself is rare.

PROBLEMS

IMPOTENCE

The most common and most disturbing sexual problem among men is the absence of erectile function. For years, the reasons for impotence were thought to be psychological—"it's all in his mind"—but the role of physical factors is becoming more and more evident as research accumulates. Alcohol is one factor that can cause problems that go beyond one night's failure. Smoking is another. Diabetes too can cause impotence, even at an early age, because the disease damages nerves and blood vessels. And owing to its commonness and complexity, impotence is the subject of a separate section of this book. (See chapter 5.)

Impotence is the most pervasive penile sexual problem that can arise, but there are others as well. Here are some:

PENILE INJURY

The erect, inflexible penis can be injured during intercourse, usually when it thrusts abruptly against a woman's pubis or pubic bone. Swelling, bleeding, impotence, and sometimes deformity of the penis can result, particularly if the injury goes untreated. In one such case, a college student literally broke off his penis in his girlfriend when she was straddling him during vigorous intercourse. As he thrust deeply into her, she suddenly fell backward, bending his erect penis inside her. Both heard a pop. The suspensory ligament of the penis was broken, causing internal bleeding. This fellow didn't go to a hospital for two days, too late for effective surgical repair. As a consequence, his penis was permanently deformed and from then on he was unable to achieve normal erections.

In addition to this sort of injury, the penile urethra also can be permanently damaged by plastic swizzle sticks, ballpoint pens, hat pins, or other objects stuck into it to stimulate sensation. Whatever the cause of injury, any penile injury should be treated by a doctor immediately.

PEYRONIE'S DISEASE

François de la Peyronie first described the functional shortening and curvature of the penis in 1743. It is a relatively common problem occurring in men ranging in age from teen years on into their eighties. Its cause remains unknown. Typically, patients are between forty-five and sixty years old. Difficult intercourse is commonly associated with this problem, but only half of patients may experience painful erections. The usual presenting sign of Peyronie's is a lump or growth on the top side of the penis. It is formed by a substance called plaque and feels like gristle.

The past few decades have yielded significant advances in the understanding of Peyronie's Disease. New noninvasive techniques and limited surgical techniques have been developed, though they should be discussed with a urologist before any procedure is attempted. Moreover, various medications may also be tried prior to more drastic surgical procedures. Vitamin E, a free radical scavenger, may offer improvement and is appropriate treatment initially in patients waiting on a decision about definitive treatment. Surgical removal of plaques has been attempted, but scarring sometimes results, with little, if any, improvement. In the most severely deformed penis, the most effective treatment may be a penile prosthesis. The good news in all of this is that this disease is still being studied and research seems to show a high incidence of spontaneous improvement in Peyronie's patients. In addition, simple reassurance helps to improve the condition, at least from a psychological standpoint: many patients immediately think cancer when they develop Peyronie's plaques in their penis, and they rest much easier when they learn that their condition is something else entirely—something that might even clear up on its own with time.

Joe, a patient of mine, provides an example of a relatively typical Peyronie's case. A fifty-five-year-old carpenter, he came in with a lump near the top of his penis. For the past three months his erections bent at that point and were painful. The erections were no longer full, but looked like an hourglass, as though blood was not getting through. When this man tried intercourse, his penis bent back on itself. Because of the lump, he feared cancer. I prescribed vitamin E, but perhaps helped most by reassuring him that the condition was not cancer and that in one-third of patients it disappears or softens without treatment. In three months his pain was gone and he could have intercourse again, but carefully, because his shaft was still bent slightly.

BALANITIS

Balanitis is an inflammation of and tightness in the foreskin and underlying tissues at the head of the penis, where, in uncircumcised men, a natural secretion called smegma can collect. The condition can be caused by friction from damp clothing, chemicals in clothing fabrics, or a reaction to various contraceptives. Some men are allergic to vaginal jellies and creams or to lubricants in condoms. The effect is a reddening and irritation of the penis. The easiest solution in these cases is to change jellies or condoms. Other cases may be relieved with salves, but there are also cases, such as recurrent infection, when the only remedy is circumcision, which can be performed on an outpatient basis with local anesthetic.

John, a thirty-eight-year-old teacher, complained of recurring inflammation on the head of his penis, as well as of tight foreskin, which he had treated in the past with salves. His problem was resolved by a circumcision, performed under local anesthetic. This was a case where circumcision for hygienic purposes was appropriate. Recurrent problems with infection, such as with this patient, who was also diabetic, require surgery.

PHIMOSIS

This condition makes it difficult to retract a tightened foreskin off the penile head: the hood, so to speak, won't go up. It's caused by chronic infection that makes the foreskin trap bacteria, though it may be congenital as well. Circumcision may be necessary for cure. That was the diagnosis for Sam, a sixty-seven-year-old lawyer who obviously didn't believe in yearly checkups. On a visit to be checked for phimosis, he told me he hadn't seen the head of his penis for years. Upon examination, I found his uncircumcised penis foul-smelling and inflamed, so much so that I could not pull the foreskin back to examine the head. Circumcision was necessary to relieve the conditions—and in that process I found a cancer.

PARAPHIMOSIS

Caused by infection or trauma, paraphimosis prevents a tightened foreskin from going back over the head of the penis. It is stuck behind the head, becoming tightened like a constricting ring around the penis and produces swelling. The swelling can be rather substantial and quite painful, as it was for Paul, a thirty-eight-year-old realtor, who appeared in my office with a gigantic, swollen penis, his foreskin having gotten stuck behind the head of his uncircumcised penis dur-

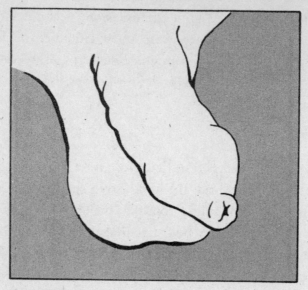

Phimosis

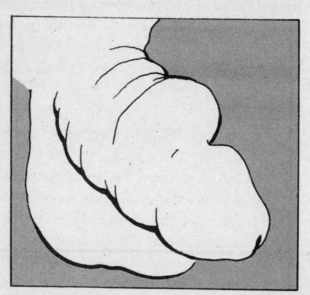

Paraphimosis with edema

ing what he claimed was an "afternoon business meeting" in a local motel. His penis had swollen to three or four times its normal size while he was doing business; by now it looked like a glazed doughnut. I relieved the pressure by lubricating the head of the penis and pushing it back through the ring, something like slipping a tight ring off a finger. Later I made permanent cure possible with a circumcision.

URETHRAL STRICTURE

This condition restricts urine flow via a narrowing of the urethral tube in one or several places. In concept, it is similar to a long tunnel with what appears to be a very constricted opening at the far end. A urethral stricture usually is caused by infection or trauma, but sometimes it is congenital in origin. Its signs are a slow, weak urine flow and, sometimes, weakened expulsion of seminal fluid. Urethral discharge is also a frequent symptom.

Urethral strictures may be single or multiple and may appear in various places within the urethra, anywhere from the tip of the penis to the area of the prostate. Treatment may be either dilating the tube with a special instrument or cutting it in the appropriate places with a special instrument.

PRIAPISM

The persistent erection that defines priapism might seem to be the ultimate male fantasy. It isn't: an erection that won't go away even after ejaculation is abnormal and in fact can cause permanent damage to blood vessel integrity. Priapism produces an erection even in the absence of sexual stimulation, or it maintains an erection after intercourse, because the blood engorging the penis cannot flow back by general circulation through the body. The cause usually is a red-blood-cell disease or injury to the spinal cord, but it also may follow injections to initiate erections (see Chapter 5). Priapism should be treated immediately—which means a visit to a hospital emergency room or a doctor's office. If the condition can be corrected quickly by medication or irrigation of the penis, normal erectile functions probably will be regained. Otherwise, surgery may be necessary. Even with immediate treatment, however, impotence may result from a bout of priapism.

Skin Problems

Like the owner of a new car who notices every nick and scratch, a man will examine his penis for minute aberrations. Blackheads and whiteheads can form on any part of penile skin, commonly appearing on the underside of the penis. These little devils are more of a nuisance than anything else. They are caused by plugged glands or ducts, and though they may be easily popped out, they probably will reappear. Rashes and moles likewise are common, and may cause no problems. Still, anything particularly bothersome or unusual should be checked, especially a mole that shows any changes in shape or color. A doctor can tell whether skin problems are significant, such as symptoms of balanitis, or harmless.

Drips After Urination

"No matter how you jump and dance, the last few drops go in your pants"—there is an inescapable truth in that old verse. It's a circumstance called postmicturitional dribbling, and that's the way it is.

Here's an experiment you can conduct yourself. After urinating, apply gentle upward pressure under the base of the penis. In most cases the pressure will squeeze out those last few drops.

BITES

Bites on the penis, whether from a playful sex partner or a dangerous insect, should receive prompt medical attention. Take the case of Doug, a hunter at a deer camp in the hills who was bitten on the penis while using an outhouse. At first the bite felt like a pinprick, but within hours the bite area became stiff and intensely painful. Soon the hunter experienced chills, fever, sweating, nausea, and severe abdominal pain. Fortunately, a doctor was in the camp, and he treated the victim with antivenin for what he recognized as a black widow spider bite. The hunter recovered fully.

Of more than 30,000 species of spiders in the world, fifty are known to bite humans. Two that are deadly are named by their colors, black widow and brown recluse. Both may be found in residential and recreational areas. The black widow, an aggressive spider that will attack on slight provocation, spins its web in darkened places—including outhouses.

PENILE TRAUMA

Because the penis is flexible and in a reasonably protected location, serious injuries are unusual. But they do occur. Quite common, of course, are skin injuries caused by zippers; less common but still seen is skin damage caused by applying the business end of a vacuum-cleaner tube to an erection, presumably to assist masturbation. Other injury can be caused by such obvious sources as missiles, bullets, knives, blunt instruments, and burns, and such unconventional sources as a chain saw or the power takeoff (unprotected drive shaft) on a hay machine.

Much of the time, such trauma can be successfully treated. On a trip to Bangkok, I learned of a unique case of penile injury and repair. A soldier's ex-wife had severed his penis, and surgeons replaced it with a penis that was removed from a transsexual during a sex-change operation. The replacement penis grew into its new place nicely, and it had the added benefit of greatly improving its new owner's outlook on his future. As far as I know, the operation was the world's first penile transplant.

FOREIGN BODIES

Young men, especially preteen boys, experiment with their erections and consequently appear in emergency rooms with a bewildering array of objects stuck inside. I have removed pencils, pens, hat pins, and straight pins from inside young penises. In one extreme case a fifteen-year-old boy inserted a pencil up his urethra while masturbating, and the next thing he knew the pencil was gone. An X ray found the pencil in the bladder. I removed it through the normal channel—the way it went in.

Penile injuries can result from various other experimentation, too. Emergency-room physicians occasionally must remove rings that were rolled onto a penis in its relaxed state and then stuck tight after erection when blood could not escape. Among the bizarre objects I have seen hanging from a penis is a monkey wrench; the patient's penis was trapped by the hole in the handle.

CHAPTER FOUR

THE TESTICLES

Testicles (also known as testes) are an obvious and sensitive part of a man's sex system. They are the source of sperm—the seed of life itself—and of a male hormone, testosterone, to which we owe such masculine effects as facial hair and deep voices. And although they are conspicuous, at least in the locker room, they are usually not a source of self-consciousness, as penis size may be. Each testicle is about two inches long and a bit more than an inch wide, and even a casual look reveals that one hangs lower than the other. Nobody knows why, but the difference is perfectly normal. Neither is there reason for concern when one testicle is slightly larger or smaller than the other, which is actually quite common. Size does not affect function. Neither, in fact, does number: a man can live quite nicely with just one testicle, be the other lost via an accident or an operation or absent at birth, as sometimes happens. With one testicle, a man's sperm and hormone production can be normal and he need have no related concerns about performing sexually or fathering children. In each testicle there are two types of cells where elements essential to sexual functioning are manufactured. One type manufactures sperm, while the other creates testosterone.

A sperm cell carries a man's genetic material, which, when combined with that in the female's egg at fertilization, creates a new life. Sperm swim through the reproductive channels of the male and later the female by swishing their tails back and forth. The testicles produce sperm in astronomical numbers, literally billions every year, although only one single sperm is needed for reproduction. Unlike women, who cease ovulation (the release of eggs) after menopause, men produce sperm continually throughout life, from puberty on. If sperm aren't released through ejaculation, they die in the productive chain and are absorbed by the body, but they are continually replaced.

After being produced in seminiferous tubes in the testicle, sperm cells move slowly through the epididymis, a microscopic network of coils behind the testicle. The trip takes about ninety days, the length of the sperm maturation process. Having matured, sperm cells swim through another tube, the vas deferens, pairs of which run from the testicle along and behind the bladder. These join at the seminal vesicles, pairs of glands that produce seminal fluid. Sperm is ejaculated, with semen, from the prostate, through the urethral tube in the penis.

The presence and potency of sperm can be determined by means of a fertility test. Such tests are usually requested after a couple has been unable to achieve pregnancy after a year or so. Computer evaluation of a laboratory sample of semen can determine quantitatively the volume, density, and motility of sperm, all factors in fertility. Two or three analyses over six to eight weeks usually are necessary to establish a correct pattern. Some men may be concerned about whether their underwear might affect their fertility. There is some validity in this. Snug shorts, in addition to creating the occasional uncomfortable entanglement, draw the testicles closer to the body, raising internal testicle temperature slightly. This change can reduce sperm count and, in some men, impact fertility.

Testosterone hormones are produced by Leydig's cells, another type of testicular cell. Upon being produced, testosterone immediately enters the bloodstream for distribution throughout the body, where it serves a number of purposes: testosterone is essential for sperm production and influences sexual aggression, sexual attraction, ability to obtain an erection, and potency. Unlike sperm production, production of testosterone diminishes with age after peaking in the late teens.

It is estimated that more than two hundred hormones are produced in the human body. Of all these, testosterone is known as the male hormone because of its exclusively male functions; estrogen is the analogous female hormone because of its influence on ovulation and its role in maintaining the condition of the vagina. Actually, each of these hormones are produced by both sexes, though in appropriately proportionate quantities.

The covering of the testicles, what shows outside, is the scrotum, a sack with a compartment for each testicle. These compartments are separated by a septum, which acts as a fire wall, helping to control temperature. The scrotum's most important function is protection of the testicles and temperature control. Testicles are cooler than the rest of the body by one or two degrees, a temperature more favorable for the manufacture of sperm. Muscles in the scrotum walls delicately control temperature by raising the testicles (moving them closer to the body) when outside temperatures are cool and lowering them when outside temperature is warmer. The spermatic cord, to which each testicle is attached like a yo-yo, also plays a role in temperature control, as its muscles help in this movement. In combination, they're a built-in climate-control system. Scrotal muscles also tighten at times of sexual arousal, perhaps as a protective device to lessen the possibility of damage in close contact.

The up-front position of the testicles makes self-examination simple, and periodic examination is a good habit to develop. The best time to examine is while taking a warm shower or bath because the scrotum is relaxed at those times. Each testicle should feel like a hard-boiled egg with the shell removed. There should be no hard spots or lumps. Evidence of even painless lumps that feel hard should be reported to a physician immediately.

Two stories from my clinical experience illustrate the value of self-examination. Early one Saturday morning, I received a phone call from my longtime friend Tom. In a distinctly frightened voice, he said he had three balls. I told him that it wasn't possible. To relieve his anxiety, we met at my office. An examination revealed that Tom had a spermatocele, a benign growth located alongside his normal testicle, and it did look like a third testicle. These growths are usually noted on self-examination, and need only to be observed periodically. If they become painful, enlarge rapidly, or become bothersome, they can be surgically removed. I told Tom that the growth wouldn't go away by itself but that it was nothing to worry about and there was no need to operate. It's still there, a year later. I told Tom we might pick up some easy change betting we had five balls between us, but he failed to enjoy my humor.

Not all stories are so lighthearted. Bob, a graduate student, had read about testicular self-examination. He tried it and found a pea-sized bump on his right testicle. Two days later, he was in my office. I saw right away that the growth was cancerous and removed it the next day. There were no signs that it had spread. This was a case where self-examination found a cancer early, so a cure was possible.

All of the conditions described in the following paragraphs are abnormalities of the testicles and indicate a need to see a doctor:

Undescended testicles   Normally, testicles develop within the abdomen and descend just before birth or soon afterward. If one has descended improperly or incompletely, repair should be made by early childhood.

Twisted testicles   Normally, a testicle hangs from the spermatic cord like the clapper of a bell. Twisting and untwisting, or intermittent torsion on the cord, can occur during normal physical activity or even while sleeping, causing pain. The result of an anatomical defect, this condition most often occurs in young males, but not exclusively. Emergency surgery is recommended if the cord does not untwist.

Varicoceles   In this condition, veins in the spermatic cord enlarge and under examination feel like a bag of worms. The

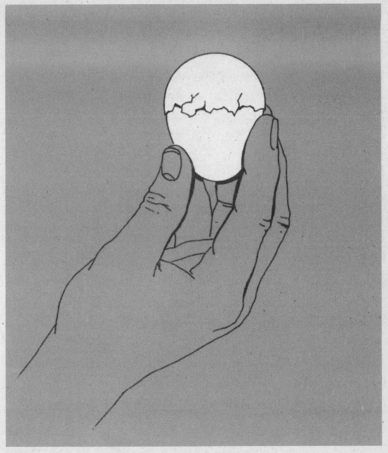

A normal testicle should feel like a hard-boiled egg without the shell.

condition is common in the mid-teens and usually is felt near the left testicle and cord. The bag of worms usually collapses when the patient is lying down. The feeling is uncomfortable, and the presence of varicoceles sometimes can cause a low sperm count, and treatment may thus be called for if infertility is an issue.

Inguinal hernia   A rupture on the side of the spermatic cord in the groin causes a bulge that is most visible when a man has been standing for quite a while. It may be painful and can strangulate bowels if trapped. The swelling usually abates or disappears when the patient is lying down.

Appendix testis   This is a small growth normally attached to the testicle that can become inflamed or twisted, causing severe pain, tenderness, and swelling. Surgical removal is the usual cure.

Hydrocele   A collection of fluid surrounding the testicle, a hydrocele makes the scrotum feel like a water balloon. The size varies with the volume of fluid. This condition can usually be diagnosed with a flashlight and remedied by a simple surgical excision if it becomes bothersome.

Epididymitis   An inflammation of the epididymis caused by bacteria or virus, epididymitis causes swelling and pain that often are accompanied by fever and chills. These are tender, hot balls.

Spermatocele   A spermatocele is a cystic, grapelike mass containing enlarged sperm tubes near the epididymis. Though not cancerous, spermatoceles often cause concern because they are abnormal growths.

Orchitis   Inflammation of the testicles that produces painful swelling, orchitis usually is associated with mumps, sometimes with epididymitis. Shrinkage of the testicles may occur after the disease clears.

Cancer   Most tumors of the testicle are cancerous, and most develop between the ages of fifteen and forty. Testicular cancer is relatively rare in other age groups. A testicle with a cancerous tumor is hard and may be swollen, but the lump or swelling usually is painless. Most testicular lumps and abnormalities are discovered by self-examination, any abnormality should be reported to a doctor immediately. Ninety percent of testicular cancers can be cured.

CHAPTER FIVE

IMPOTENCE

Impotence, the inability to achieve an erection and follow through with normal intercourse, occurs with surprising frequency as men age. An estimated 10 million men in the United States are either permanently or situationally impotent, though probably less than 10 percent of these patients ever actually visits a physician for their problem. Almost every man at some point in his life experiences temporary, or situational, impotence due to any of an assortment of causes; common culprits include too much to drink, mental preoccupation, and lack of interest from or in a partner. This inhibition is easily explained and soon overcome. Lasting impotence is caused by more complex factors.

Until recently, impotence was blamed almost exclusively on psychological issues. In the 1960s and 1970s, for instance, doctors thought mental concerns were responsible for 95 percent of impotence cases. The remaining 5 percent were attributed to evident physical causes such as obvious nerve damage. Now, however, doctors believe the cause of impotence is as likely to be physical as psychological. This shift is based on better diagnostic methods and on discoveries made possible by more sophisticated means of measuring physical and chemical changes, particularly in the vascular field and in the study of diabetes. Much of this progress may be attributed to a new interest in the scientific study of sex pioneered by Dr. Alfred Kinsey in the 1940s and 1950s. After Kinsey blazed a trail, researchers began looking where they had not looked before in all areas of human sexuality, not only impotence.

Physical as well as psychological causes of impotence may be treated and, to a considerable extent, corrected—sometimes in dramatic fashion. Following are some dominant physical and psychological causes of impotence, along with some evidence of their effects.

PHYSICAL IMPOTENCE

DRUGS

A fellow doctor found that he had become impotent and came to me for help. At the time he was treating himself for ulcers with the drug cimetidine. That was a clue, for while that drug is quite effective as a medication for ulcers, it also may lower production of the male hormone testosterone. His complaint of impotence was typical among cimetidine users. I recommended a substitute medication, and the impotence problem disappeared.

Chemicals are the most common physical cause of impotence. Other medications—legal and otherwise—with side effects related to impotence include high–blood pressure pills (antihypertensives), which impact the blood pressure necessary for an erection; recreational drugs such as marijuana, ecstasy, cocaine, and amphetamines, which affect the central nervous system; antihistamines, such as cold pills; tranquilizers; weight-loss pills; diuretics; and sedatives.

Alcohol abuse is another frequently seen factor in impotence, and it can have a more lasting impact than one night's disappointment. Nicotine too, from cigarette smoking, can cause impotence by constricting small blood vessels and limiting blood supply to the penis as well as to elsewhere throughout the body.

Abnormal Blood Pressure

A retired insurance executive, age seventy, complained that his capacity to achieve an erection had been diminished after a coronary bypass operation and he could never get hard enough for penetration. He said, rather colorfully, that attempting intercourse was like trying to put an oyster in a parking meter. His problem was permanently decreased blood flow. When a trial of Viagra was not completely satisfactory, the best solution was implantation of a penile prosthesis—an artificial stiffener.

Because blood rushes into the penis to create an erection, obstruction of the blood vessels can result in impotence. High blood pressure, hardening of the arteries, Peyronie's disease, and diabetes are among the diseases that can clog the erectile fuel line. A technique for measuring blood pressure in the penis also can confirm whether pressure there is abnormally low among some men.

Nerve Impulse Abnormalities

A forty-two-year-old man suffering from diabetes was also suffering from a sex problem too embarrassing, he thought, to take to a doctor in his own city so he traveled two hundred miles to consult me: he had not had an erection for more than a year, but he could ejaculate while masturbating, which he did, often with his wife's participation. As it turned out, his diabetes had speeded his aging process and in so doing affected both his nerves and his blood vessels. We worked together to control his diabetes and used the new drug Viagra with very successful treatment and results.

Perhaps as instructive too is the case of a thirty-two-year-old professional bicyclist who complained of numbness and tingling in his penis and impotence after a 350-mile bicycle race. The culprit was his hard and narrow bicycle seat, which put pressure on the blood vessels and nerves to his penis. The problem resolved with rest and no bike riding for a while.

As may be seen via this case, nerves that control the penis are as essential to an erection as is blood. Diseases that can reduce or interrupt critical nerve impulses include strokes, spinal-cord injuries, kidney disease, diabetes, and alcoholism. Nerve injuries from abdominal or pelvic surgery, or other causes, also inhibit nerve functions.

HORMONAL ABNORMALITIES

Impotence is rarely caused by an imbalance of hormones, but kidney and liver diseases, kidney dialysis, and alcoholism can adversely affect normal hormone balance. Such was the circumstance for Richard, a fifty-nine-year-old impotent patient of mine, who was found to have a very low level of testosterone—the result of a disease of the liver called hemochromatosis. The proper testosterone level was restored by injections. He eventually did get erections and declared an increase in his sexual desire.

PSYCHOLOGICAL IMPOTENCE

DEPRESSION

Mental depression can tax a man's sex drive as well as his energy. Inability to achieve an erection leads to further depression and thus a vicious cycle. One clue that the root of impotence may be psychological is the presence of involuntary nocturnal erections. Take the case of Nick: A security guard, Nick had not wanted a divorce, but his wife left him for his best friend and took her and Nick's four children with her. After she left, Nick's depression deepened and his potency failed altogether. He visited a psychiatrist regularly for a year, after which he felt more at ease psychologically but still got no help in getting an erection. Things looked up when Nick found a new girlfriend and dated her for a year that included a delightful trip to Hawaii. Nevertheless, she left him because he was incapable of getting an erection.

When he came to me, at age fifty, he had been divorced for three years and no longer had a girlfriend. His routine included weekly visits to a massage parlor for fellatio, which brought him to ejaculation, but without erection. However, he did awaken with a morning piss hard-on, so I was able to convince him that his erection mechanism still worked and that he was suffering not from anything physical but from depression and performance anxiety. Happily, he got well in time.

STRESS

Rory, a forty-four-year-old travel agent, was typical of many patients. He was considering divorce, a possibility enthusiastically encouraged by a new girlfriend. She was much younger than he, and he hoped to impress her—but probably more himself—with his passionate bedroom performance. He soon found he was no longer the sexual sensation that he remembered being in his younger years, though. He forgot that the brain is a sex organ, the biggest of them all, and he was bombarding it with visions that were more than he could handle. Problems with job, marriage, or money can easily become problems with sex. Inability to get an erection provokes stress, and a vicious cycle ensues.

PERFORMANCE ANXIETY

Performance anxiety can stem from any number of factors. Greg, a lawyer, could gain an erection and have intercourse with his alcoholic wife, but he didn't enjoy it. He instead chose to take a paramour to his mountain cabin. However, the secluded location, the fireside, the soft music, and the wind in the trees unfortunately did him no good: he couldn't get an erection. He tried different women, the same cabin, the same romantic accessories, and still no erection. He confided that he felt like somebody was trying to tell him something; I suggested he go to a marriage counselor. He did and the counselor did tell him something: Go back to your wife. His wife, too, went to a counselor for alcoholism therapy. They're back on a one-way street, working hard at their relationship.

A similar problem afflicted a forty-five-year-old fellow

who successfully lured a lady to bed the night he met her but was embarrassed because he couldn't get an erection no matter how hard both tried. He apologized, saying he guessed that he was over the hill. The attitude and condition improved substantially, however, when he and his new friend got to know each other better and were more relaxed. Both Greg's case and this latter well illustrate performance anxiety: each man was feeling pressure—here evidently from psyches telling them they should not perhaps be doing what they were doing—manifested in an inability to achieve erection.

Other men, such as Jack, a twenty-eight-year-old bricklayer, have other issues. Jack could have normal intercourse except when he tried to put on a condom. Each time he tried to roll a rubber onto his penis, his erection faded. It was obvious to me that Jack had a psychological problem related to condom use.

Persistent failure to achieve an erection, for whatever reason, can become self-perpetuating. Fear of failure is reinforced by failure and can even turn into expectation of failure.

MISINFORMATION

A young man came in with a problem many men would like to have: he could make love to his girlfriend once a night easily, but he thought he should be able to do it three or four times. Was something wrong?

Well, there *was* something missing if this fellow wanted to be like the pro football player who bragged that he could make it with five women a day, except on game days. But for mere mortals, once a night consistently is average.

Misinformation about sex begins as soon as boys are old enough to discover there are differences between boys and girls. It takes adult forms, too, in myths about how a real man should perform, how a woman should react, how hope is lost with old age. Most men aren't as "real" as they'd like to believe they are, and worse, like cars, they peter out as time progresses.

Getting the facts straight is a serious matter. Take this example: Statistics show that men who have had coronary bypass surgery are more likely to resume normal sexual activity than are men who have had heart attacks. Evidence indicates that this may be because the partner of the heart attack victim is apprehensive about another attack. Yet some cardiologists say that if a man can climb a flight of stairs, he can safely have sex. So, heart attack patients and their partners should get the proper information from their doctors, because they might needlessly be missing out on a normal sex life. Others would be wise to follow suit: Knowledge is power.

Schemes or devices to overcome impotence are as old as history. Potions have been drunk, gods have been invoked, lotions have been applied, witchcraft has been employed, honey and spices have been blended—all for the purpose of producing impressive erections. Stimulants, or hoped-for stimulants, have ranged from carrots and peas, parsnips, and herbs to powdered animal horns and ground-up genitals. The world's rhinoceros population, in fact, was almost wiped out because of a number of Asian cultures' belief in the aphrodisiac powers of powdered rhino horns. (This belief still exists among some people, and poachers still kill rhinos for horns worth $1,000 apiece. The danger of extinction of the endangered animals remains very real.)

Furthermore, man's search for foolproof sexual fulfillment has literally covered the globe, in the vain hope that there were some particular place where sexual shortcomings could be cured. Ponce de Leon, for instance, discovered Florida while in search of a fabled fountain of youth, which meant just one thing: eternal potency.

Today medical science has found answers to impotence—and while we stay closer to home, we're still turning to potions and powders and devices. Now, however, we call them medications and they are quite practical, not to mention scientifically proven reliable. The number-one medication in the twentieth century, for example, was Viagra (sildenafil citrate), which made its debut on March 27, 1998, when the Food and Drug Administration announced that the diamond-shaped blue pill was available for treatment of impotence of various types. Other modalities for treating impotence include penile injections and penile prostheses, which are surgically implanted devices. Of course, a patient should consult a urologist before embarking on *any* treatment for impotence.

First let us talk about Viagra. Before its introduction to the public, it went through numerous randomized, placebo-controlled trials involving more than three thousand men with various degrees of impotence stemming from such diverse causes as diabetes, spinal-cord injury, and history of prostate surgery, as well as patients with no identifiable organic cause of impotence. These patients also suffered a wide range of other illnesses, including hypertension, coronary-artery disease and diabetes. In the trials, the men using Viagra® reported success more often than those using a placebo, and the rates of success increased with dose. Further, the findings were consistent in men representing a wide variety of causes for erectile dysfunction or impotence.

Before the introduction of Viagra, medically legitimate options for impotence sufferers centered on a limited, invasive, and expensive range of treatments including surgically inserted penile implants, vacuum pumps, injections of vasoactive drugs, and suppositories inserted into the penis by way of the urethra. Viagra is the first oral treatment ever approved for impotence and by far the most natural way to treat this disorder. It works by simply boosting the chemicals involved in the natural process of erection, allowing the user to respond naturally to sexual stimulation. If there is no sexual stimulation, Viagra does nothing. If there is sexual stimulation, an erection occurs in most patients. Hence, the patient certainly has more control over the erection than he would with vasoactive drugs, with which an erection is triggered immediately upon injection and is sometimes inconvenient.

As far as side effects from Viagra, mild headache, flushing, nasal stuffiness, some stomachache, and mild and temporary changes in perception of color and light have been reported. Most healthy men can take Viagra, although it is not recommended for men who are currently taking nitroglycerine, as the combination may lower the blood pressure below acceptable levels.

As a urologist, I treat and have treated a wide variety of men. All of them want to live and love to the fullest of their ability, and no matter how much one tries, it is very difficult to ignore that physiologic process. Impotence can rob a man of his ability to express this urge which is so important for his well being. Unfortunately, with age comes a slower, weaker sexual response and a decreasing ability to sustain an erection long enough for sex. It is precisely because Viagra can help all of the problems of the aging, be they incurred by prostate surgery, spinal-cord injury, diabetes, or vascular difficulties, that it is hailed as a wonder drug.

For whatever reason, though, Viagra may not be for every man. Other options are available. The erector injector is a drug that will cause the penis to become erect for from one and a half to three hours, long enough to sustain intercourse. It is a treatment for impotence, and has been effective with about 80 percent of the men on whom it has been used. The drug is vasoactive, meaning it works on blood vessels, and is available only by prescription. It has been effective for patients with diabetes, heart or neurological problems, and for those who have had radical prostate surgery.

The patient himself injects the drug directly into his penis. The process is becoming more acceptable, though it does present certain disadvantages: instruction and counseling by a physician are required, and inexperienced patients could place the injection in the wrong place and scar the penis. Also, it is generally recommended that the injection-type therapy be used no more than twice a week. Another interesting complication is that an injection erection may not fade after a few hours, in which case an emergency call to a doctor is in order. Although it is somewhat expensive, the erector injector is less expensive than surgical implantation of a penile prosthesis.

Mechanical devices are also an option for impotence sufferers. Constriction devices, including ones utilized in conjunction with vacuums, are being more widely used by patients who are not surgical candidates or who refuse surgery, or for whom medications such as Viagra are not an option. These apparatuses either block the outflow of blood from the penis, constricting blood vessels at the base of the penis, or, in the vacuum type, draw blood into the penis, trapping it once it is there. These devices should be used only as frequently as advised by the manufacturer.

Implants—of which there are several kinds—employ artificial tubes called penile prostheses that are inserted into the penis to do the work of natural tubes (corpora cavernosa) which ordinarily fill with blood to create an erection. They fit precisely into the chambers and fill them completely. These prostheses have been developed within the past twenty-five years, and with success their use has expanded dramatically. Thousands are in use in the United States and around the world.

These prostheses fall into two basic categories: Solid tubes, in pairs, are made of silicone rubber with or without metal inserts (not enough metal to set off an airport detector). The implants remain rigid all the time, providing a perpetual erection as large and full as a normal erection. This has the advantage of preparedness but the disadvantage of being difficult to conceal in clothing. Some carry five- or ten-year guarantees!

Inflatable prostheses also come in two types. Both use hollow cylinders that may be inflated to erect positions by pumping up a self-contained sterile fluid. In one type, fluid, reservoir, and pump all are carried within the cylinders them-

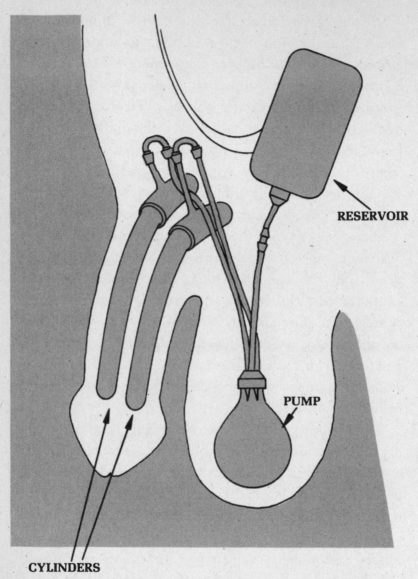

RESERVOIR

PUMP

CYLINDERS

Penile implant

selves; erection is achieved by working the cylinder pumps. In the other type, fluid is held in a reservoir implanted in the abdomen and is forced through a network of silicone tubing into the cylinders by operating a pump implanted in the scrotum.

Implant operations for both solid and inflatable prostheses are now relatively routine. In fact, the solid implant procedure may be performed on an outpatient basis. In either case, sexual relations must be suspended until approved by a doctor, usually after four to six weeks. Other than slight, quickly disappearing postoperative discomfort, implants are popular and men using them have few complaints.

Consider Charlie, who as a hotel night clerk often had time to contemplate his woes and the fact that he wasn't getting any younger. His troubles began (or, more specifically, his sex life ended) with a cancer operation four or five years earlier. He read about penile prostheses, came in to see me to further investigate, and ultimately decided to have one implanted.

He did nicely. I didn't see him again for a few weeks, but when we did meet I saw a very different Charlie. He was nattily attired and sporting a new hairstyle topped off with a jaunty tam; he had a spring in his step and a glint in his eye. The psychological change was jarring: Charlie wasn't the same man. He was a guy on the make, and there was no doubt about why. He boasted that he had recently "entertained" a lady friend and while making love to her for forty-five minutes, brought her to the first climax of her life. His prosthesis had given him a self-confidence he'd never had, even before his cancer operation.

CHAPTER SIX

THE PROSTATE GLAND

Unique to men, the prostate gland is a critical component in the ejaculation process. Yet even to men, this small gland's function is obscure—particularly when one considers that a man can function without one—its location vague, and its name often mispronounced (it's *prostate*, not *prostrate*). In fact, the prostate is uniquely suited to perform its critical male functions by virtue of its muscular composition and location immediately below the bladder, surrounding the tube that directs urine flow into the penis.

The muscular function of the prostate, coordinated with muscles in the bladder, opens and closes the tube through which urine flows from the bladder to the penis. It also helps shut off urine at the bladder, permitting semen to enter the penis during periods of sexual arousal leading to ejaculation. The tube that carries both urine and semen through the penis is the urethra. Urine and semen cannot flow through the urethra at the same time. The prostate and bladder, with help from the brain and other stimuli, determine which it shall be. The glandular function of the prostate is to manufacture a component of the semen—that sticky, milky fluid that spurts from the penis during sexual orgasm. These separate functions of the prostate are known and well understood. But there is much still unknown about the prostate's role and functions.

The prostate grows to its normal size, about the size of a walnut, at puberty, and enlarges again at about the age of fifty, a normal expansion related to aging. However, the prostate can expand well beyond its normal dimensions—in some cases it can grow as big as a grapefruit—for reasons that are not clear but are probably hormonal. Such excessive growth, called adenoma, does not involve normal prostate cells but different tissue—connective tissue, muscle, and stroma. As adenoma grows, it spreads inward and gradually applies increasing pressure to the urethra, like a squeeze valve. When the urethra is partially pinched off, signs of prostate problems appear. Symptoms are many, almost all of them having to do with urination. Here are some principal symptoms:

- Difficulty in urinating
- Changes in urinary habits, particularly more frequent urination at night
- Pain or a burning sensation while urinating
- Presence of blood in urine
- Irregular urine flow—a stream that starts, stops, stammers, and starts again
- Difficulty in stopping urine flow
- Persistent presence of dribbles that leave embarrassing spots on clothing

What's more, urination problems in the prostate can lead to related problems in other organs. For example, restricted urine flow in the prostate can put greater demands on the bladder and kidneys. This could lead to bladder infection and, if unattended, ultimately to kidney obstruction and failure. Another sign of potential prostate problems is pain that is not related to urination but is felt in other places. Pain in the lower back, pelvic region, or perineum is normal from time to time, but any pain that increases in frequency or intensity should be regarded as a warning. (The perineum is the area between the scrotum and the anus, that place most likely to be pinched by a small, narrow, or hard bicycle seat.)

Naturally, the earlier an enlarged prostate is detected, the greater the chance that it can be successfully treated. The body provides some help in detection and treatment because symptoms generally appear after age fifty and the prostate itself is relatively easy to examine. From an external perspective, the gland can be examined via the rectum, as it is located just inside the anus. In a routine digital (finger-wave) examination, a doctor can feel the prostate to test for irregularities or asymmetry in size and texture, which should be rubbery. The doctor's examination with a gloved, lubricated finger is painless and for most patients is only slightly uncomfortable. The examination is limited, however, because the doctor can feel only the back side of the gland.

A new technique, called transrectal ultrasonography, can obtain more information about the prostate and may prove to be more effective in early detection of prostate cancer, which now is very hard to find in early stages. Ultrasonography uses sonar, via a small probe inserted into the rectum, sound impulses are projected back and forth across the prostate at controlled depths, working back layer after layer

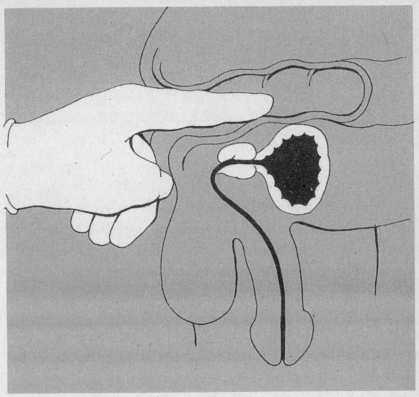

"Finger wave," or digital rectal examination, by way of the rectum to feel the prostate for problems such as cancer. Routine prostate examination should be performed at yearly intervals after the age of forty.

and registering the reflected images on a screen like a TV set. The ultrasound machine usually is operated by a urologist, a specialist who deals with urinary-tract problems in men and women, and to whom a personal physician refers his patient if abnormalities are suspected. Although promising, however, transrectal ultrasound examination of the prostate is not yet a proven prostate-cancer screening technique. It does aid in guiding biopsy needles to suspicious areas of the prostate, but future studies are needed to determine its real potential.

PROSTATE PROBLEMS

Benign Prostatic Hyperplasia ("Old Man's Disease")

Fred, a sixty-seven-year-old retired lumber broker, was getting up four to five times every night to urinate. He came to see me partly because he was worried, but mostly because his wife was worried as well as tired of being awakened by his frequent night calls. Sometimes Fred's urine flow was normal, but at other times he was slow to start and slow to finish. He also felt the need to go again as soon as he got back in bed, but return trips produced very little. He said he had cut down on drinking, thinking that it might have had something to do with his condition, but this didn't help much. He also told me that his father and two older brothers had had prostate operations. He wanted to know if prostate conditions were hereditary, and I told him that we really don't know.

Then Fred and I discussed a transurethral resection, a relatively simple operation—in fact, the least complicated of prostate operations—to clear obstructive tissue from his prostate. Fred decided to go this route and I performed the procedure, and after a while Fred's urinating returned to normal. Now he gets up only once a night, some nights not at all.

Fred's condition was benign prostatic hyperplasia, an apparent overproduction of cells within the prostate gland. Growth of adenoma tissue extends inward toward the urethra and in time can restrict urine flow and block the tube. (A patient who was a logger described his condition nicely when he said, "Doc, I can't strip the bark off the tree anymore.")

Benign prostatic hyperplasia (BPH) affects about one-third of men over age fifty, more than half of men in their sixties, and as many as 90 percent of men in their seventies and eighties. The prostate itself has two primary growth periods—one during puberty and the next starting about the age of twenty-five. During this second growth period, the prostate may press against the urethra, acting like a hose clamp. Secondarily, the bladder wall can become irritated, and as a result contract when containing only a small amount of urine, this leading to frequent urination. Eventually, if left untreated, the bladder may weaken and lose its ability to empty fully. Then, urine remains in the bladder after apparent voiding, or more seriously, one can also go into urinary retention or total stoppage if the bladder fails to initiate urination or to empty itself at all.

In addition to urination difficulties, some patients may experience pain with urination, or find blood in their urine but experience no pain. Symptoms of this sort should be reported immediately to a doctor. There are many treatment options for benign prostatic hyperplasia. Be sure to carefully discuss what might be best for you with your urologist or physician before deciding on what course you would like to try.

ACUTE PROSTATITIS ("FIRE BELOW")

Roger, a twenty-eight-year-old professional basketball player, was overcome during a practice session with what seemed to be a sudden attack of flu. He had alternate chills and fever, muscular aches and pains all over, and discomfort in his lower back and perineum. He had to urinate frequently, and urination was very painful. At times his stream was pink, as if tinted with blood.

Finding Roger's prostate gland tender and swollen, the team physician sent him to me. I diagnosed acute prostatitis, a urinary-tract infection (it was, in fact, blood that Roger was seeing), and prescribed antibiotics and rest. Within a few days Roger felt only mild discomfort, and within a week he was back on the court. A follow-up examination revealed no further infection.

Acute prostatitis is an infection of the prostate gland caused by bacteria. It can occur in any man from adolescence to old age, and it often hits suddenly. Symptoms usually are a combination of urinary difficulties (as in hyperplasia) and nausea, chills, fever, vomiting, and aches and pains (as in influenza). Antibiotic drugs and rest are an effective treatment.

Chronic Prostatitis ("Pain Near the Ass")

One day in the men's locker room, I ran into Malcolm, an engineer who plays golf where I do. He confided in me that he was having urinary-tract symptoms—the same symptoms that he had experienced every year or so for the last fifteen years. He had to urinate more often than usual, and felt a burning sensation each time he did. I suggested he come to see me at my office.

Telling me more when he came for his consultation, he said he didn't have chills or fever and saw no blood in his urine. Nevertheless, tests indicated a urinary-tract infection, which I found to be low-grade prostatitis. Fortunately, treat-

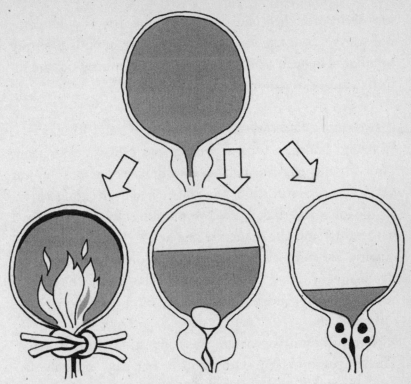

Three things can happen to your prostate: Prostatitis, *left*, feels like a fire, with urination frequency, burning, constriction, and possible bleeding caused by infection in most cases. Benign prostatic hyperplasia, *center*, is a normal benign growth that occurs with aging; the cause is unknown and symptoms include slow stream (flow), incomplete emptying, and urinary "blockage." Cancer, *right*, is also of an unknown cause; there may be no apparent symptoms present.

ment was simple: antibiotics and a warm bath two or three times a day. He was still able to play golf, but the prescribed treatment took priority over teeing off.

Stress is frequently associated with chronic prostatitis, with or without a urinary-tract infection. It is a condition that professional men and business executives in high-stress jobs seem prone to acquire. So do truck drivers, who combine the stress of freeway driving with long periods of sitting in a bouncing cab. Antibiotics or urinary antiseptics are effective means of treatment.

Congestive Prostatitis ("Nothing Spells Relief")

Reverend Smith, a forty-eight-year-old celibate clergyman, came in with pains in two hard-to-describe areas. One was perineal, which made him feel as if he had been riding a bicycle too long, and the other was suprapubic, which gave him a pain right below the navel. He said he also had to urinate frequently. He confided that he had occasional discharges, usually white or clear, from his penis. He had no history of venereal disease, and no outlet for sex except occasional masturbation.

Reverend Smith's problem was congestion of the prostate. The congestion is caused by semen that clogs the tube because it hasn't been ejaculated. Frequent, urgent calls to urinate, often resulting in disappointing dribbles, are reported by males from adolescence on, particularly among single men and married men who are separated. Stress and other factors might be cited, but the clearly evident cause is a lack of sex. Doctors may prescribe sitz baths, massage, or antibiotics, but the truth is that masturbation usually will clear the pipeline, just as a good blow will clear a stuffed-up nose.

Hematospermia ("Rusty Pipes")

Marvin, a retired accountant, aged sixty-seven, found blood on his pajamas one morning, just a few days after his wife reported blood in her vaginal discharge after having intercourse. A methodical man, Martin determined who was doing the bleeding. Through masturbation, he found himself responsible—his seminal fluid contained specks about the size and color of coffee grounds. After this he came to me. He had no pain, no blood in his urine, no other symptoms of hyperplasia. A complete urologic examination was normal. I told him not to worry, and come back in a year.

Bloody come—evidence of blood in ejaculate—is an alarming discovery for any man. The alarm can be compounded if his partner also finds blood coming from her body after intercourse. What's happening usually is nothing worse than an inflammation of the prostate gland or seminal vesicles, which leaves traces of blood in semen. Or it could be that the excitement of intercourse and the fervor of ejaculation caused the eruption of a small blood vessel in one person or the other. The way to determine which person is bleeding is to do what Marvin did—masturbate and see. Signs in the ejaculate usually appear in one of two shades, dark specks that resemble coffee grounds, or bright red stains. It is unusual for cancer to cause such bleeding, although bloody come is most likely to occur at a time of maximum vulnerability to cancers of the prostate and bladder.

CANCER OF THE PROSTATE (SERIOUS BUSINESS)

Ralph, a sixty-six-year-old businessman, told his internist during a routine physical that he had to get up once or twice every night to urinate. He mentioned that drinking coffee or tea after dinner made nature's demands worse, so he quit. But for all the urgency, Ralph said his urine stream had slowed down in the past few years. On examination, his internist felt a nodule in his prostate, but other than that, Ralph was completely healthy. He had no indications of infection, bleeding, or backache, and his blood tests were normal.

After he was referred to me, a prostate specific antigen (PSA) test revealed an elevated level of 8.0, and a digital rectal examination confirmed the presence of a small nodule on the right side of his prostate, which his primary physician had discovered. Ultrasound scanning and biopsy of this nodule, as well as of other parts of his prostate, confirmed the diagnosis of cancer of the prostate—a low-grade Gleason Grade II-II cancer.

I performed a radical prostatectomy, which meant that I removed the entire prostate along with the seminal vesicles that lead to it, and reconnected the urethra directly to the bladder. Within a few weeks, Ralph returned to his regular daily routine. Eventually he was able to urinate normally, maintain erections, and have satisfactory intercourse. Yet while his cancer had been caught in time, follow-up consisting of a yearly PSA examination to make sure that his cancer stays cured is mandatory for this patient.

Not all patients are so fortunate. Don, a well-respected local banker, had not been seen by a physician in three years, since his retirement. Then he visited his family practitioner for a checkup. He had minimal prostate symptoms and no pain or urinary-tract abnormalities, but at sixty-three years of age, prostate exam was normal procedure. Digital rectal examination revealed a normal-feeling prostate from that perspective and only slight asymmetry of the prostate with no discrete nodularity. The routine PSA blood test, however, alerted his family practitioner that something might be amiss: Don's PSA was 49, while normal is 0–4. Don was referred to his urologist, and unfortunately ultrasound and needle biopsy of the prostate revealed a medium-grade carcinoma that had metastasized to the local prostate area. Unlike Ralph's contained prostate cancer, Don's prostate was locally invasive and beyond cure by the usual surgical technique.

In fact, it was too late for Don; his cancer was inoperable. As a result, he was subjected to a regimen that began with Lupron, a hormone-antagonist medication taken for three to four months, followed by conformal radiation therapy, which focuses radiation on a restricted field. And even though his bone scan was negative, Don's future is an unanswered question.

The statistics on prostate cancer are awesome. After lung cancer, it is the second-most-fatal cancer among men, responsible for nearly 40,000 deaths in the United States each year. Another 200,000 new cases are diagnosed annually as well. Its incidence increases with age and is most prevalent between ages sixty and eighty. Estimates say that 30 percent of American men over age fifty will have cancer of the prostate. Using those figures, nearly 1 in 10 men will develop prostate cancer, but only 1 in 300 (1.4 percent) die of it, because after eighty, most men will have it but will not necessarily die of it.

Patients want to know if there are ways to protect against prostate cancer, and they often ask about theories they have heard. One holds that sexual activity is a deterrent. While this always had been dismissed as wishful thinking, a recent British study has established some basis for the claim. Other theories speculate on the relationship between diet and cancer. It's all speculation; the answer is that there are no answers.

Cancer of the prostate is particularly insidious because it is difficult to detect; it reveals no identifiable signs in its early stages. It might cause obstruction, as other prostate problems do, or it might show nothing at all. By the time cancer does leave clues—serious problems with urination or persistent pain in the hip or back, for example—it may have spread beyond the prostate gland into neighboring bones, lymph nodes, and even the bloodstream.

In years past, more than 90 percent of prostate cancer cases were inoperable by the time they were first seen by a urologist. Today, however, if prostate cancer is detected early, a majority of cases—85 percent—can be cured by radical surgical removal. To help enhance the likelihood of early detection, every man with a family history, either father or first generation relative should have an annual PSA blood test and digital rectal prostate examination after the age of forty. If there is no family history of prostate cancer, a yearly prostate digital examination and PSA test is recommended beginning at age fifty.

Prostate cancer is diagnosed in a series of steps, similar to those in routine prostate exams. First, your medical history is reviewed and a physical examination of your prostate is performed. This is accompanied by a PSA test, which measures the level of prostatic specific antigen in a blood sample. PSA is a substance produced by both normal and malignant prostate cells. The amount of PSA in the blood increases when prostate cancer has spread, though some men with benign prostatic hyperplasia or prostatitis have an increased level of PSA without cancer. If an abnormality is found during the digital rectal examination or if an abnormal PSA blood test is noted, your family physician will refer you to a urologist for further testing.

The PSA blood test may prove to be this century's most valuable new tool in the early diagnosis of prostate cancer.

A second blood test, called a free-PSA, has become available as well; it can sometimes give a more accurate reading than the "old PSA." The free-PSA test helps tell the difference between benign prostate hypertrophy and cancer of the prostate: the "free" portion of the PSA test is the "good PSA" and the "complex" portion is the "bad PSA."

Make sure any PSA blood test is taken three days after your last ejaculation, as ejaculation can falsely elevate your PSA result. In addition, long-distance bike rides may elevate the test in some instances, owing to the constant pressure on the prostate by the hard, thin bicycle seat!

Further tests may include transrectal ultrasonography (ultrasound), which is recommended if an abnormality is found during a digital rectal exam or if you have an abnormal PSA blood test. To determine the presence of cancer, the urologist may also perform a biopsy, or the surgical removal of a small sample of tissue for the purpose of examination under a microscope to see if cancer cells exist. To do this, a biopsy needle is inserted through the ultrasound probe to take a sample of any suspicious area. No anesthetic is required for the biopsy, and it is not painful, but some urologists use a local anesthetic injected directly into the nerve bundles surrounding the prostate and prostate itself prior to the procedure. Should cancer be discovered, a bone scan may detect spread of cancer to your bones. If you are found to have cancer, your urologist will recommend the tests needed in your particular case.

When cancer has spread beyond the prostate, only treatment, but no cure, is possible. The options are not pleasant. One is to prescribe radiation therapy or chemotherapy; another is to administer estrogen to neutralize the dominating effect of testosterone, which fuels the growth of prostatic cancer cells. Another alternative is to remove the testicles, the source of testosterone, in order to slow the growth of cancer cells. Finally, one can choose to do nothing. Because we don't know the natural history of cancer of the prostate, confusion exists as to the best treatment, and the fact that there are many long-term survivors after hormone treatment alone adds to the mysteries surrounding this disease.

After any treatment for prostate cancer, you should continue to visit your urologist for regular checkups. Your doctor will examine you at various intervals following your treatment to make sure you are recovering properly and to determine if any future treatment is needed. Most important, during follow-up treatment, discuss any questions you have about your cancer with your urologist.

CHAPTER SEVEN

PROSTATE SURGERY AND OTHER OPTIONS

A common operation in the private-parts department removes obstructions in the prostate gland that block or impede normal urine flow. A surgical instrument called a resectoscope enters the gland and cuts away blockage, piece by piece. The operation offers a safe and completely effective solution for men who seem to have to urinate all the time, can't empty their bladders completely, or lose sleep because they must get up so often at night.

Such a procedure is the answer for the fellow who misses the best part of the ball game because he's in the rest room under the stands trying to get something going at the urinal, the fellow who can hear the excitement and can't help but notice that two men and a boy have come and gone in the next stall while he's still standing in place.

The name for this operation is transurethral resection of the prostate, or TURP. When more conservative measures including medications fail, a transurethral resection is the treatment of choice for an obstructed prostate gland. The name gives a clue to how the operation is performed. "Transurethral" means that the surgical instrument is directed through the urethra—the normal channel through the penis—to reach the prostate. This sounds gruesome, but no skin incision is necessary, hence no scarring. The surgery, as well as the postoperative period, is painless. For most patients, a hospital stay of one or two nights is all that is required.

Symptoms that bring men into the doctor's office and that ultimately lead to a TURP operation ordinarily involve problems in passing urine. These can be an urgency to urinate that forces a man to get up four or five times a night, difficulty in starting, pain during urination, inability to empty the bladder satisfactorily, a need to urinate again after having just done so, a urine flow that starts and stops, and even dribbling on one's pants.

On examination, the doctor probably will find that the prostate feels somewhat enlarged. He may be assisted in his diagnosis by an X ray of the kidneys or an ultrasound examination of the prostate. In most cases, the enlargement will stem from a condition called benign prostatic hyperplasia, an apparent overproduction of cells. The cause of hyperplasia is unknown, but the result is a growth within the prostate that crowds against the urethra. This crowding impedes or blocks flow from the bladder and creates other difficulties with urination, just as a clamp set too tight could cut off flow in a garden hose. The purpose of the transurethral resection of the prostate is to remove the obstructing growth, and it's sort of like peeling an orange from the inside but leaving the rind—the prostate—unchanged.

The resectoscope, the instrument that is inserted through the penis, is a long metal tube with an attached light, a channel for water flow, and a loop of fine wire that can be charged

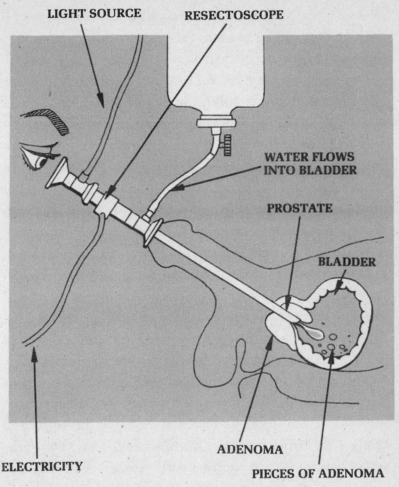

LIGHT SOURCE   **RESECTOSCOPE**

**WATER FLOWS
INTO BLADDER**

PROSTATE

BLADDER

ELECTRICITY

ADENOMA

PIECES OF ADENOMA

Transurethral resection of the prostate—a common operation for obstruction in men, done through the normal channel, or transurethrally.

with controlled amounts of electricity. The surgeon moves the loop back and forth, his hand motions akin to playing a tiny trombone, and chips away at the excess growth. The chips are irrigated out by water. The operation takes about an hour; as mentioned, it is not painful, and neither is the postoperative period. After the operation, a catheter is inserted through the prostate and into the bladder to drain blood and urine and to give the bladder a rest.

Usually, the patient can eat a normal meal on the evening after or on the morning following the operation. The catheter may be removed the following morning. Then the patient may go home, to lead a sedentary life for three to four weeks. The operation is successful in 95 percent of all cases; in a few cases, regrowth of obstructive tissues may occur. Further, it must be noted that a TURP cannot guarantee freedom from cancer; that is not its purpose. It is still possible that cancer unrelated to the operation can develop months or years later.

Urinary incontinence is not common after a transurethral resection. There may be mild leakage for a time after returning from the hospital; this usually clears up after a few weeks. And in most cases, the operation does not impede erectile function; if the patient was potent before the operation, he will usually be potent after it. However, potency should not be confused with fertility. Frequently, patients become infertile after a transurethral resection because the operation changes the structure of the bladder neck. That change diverts ejaculate from its normal path through the penis, and sends it into the bladder instead. There is no change in sensation, but at the moment of orgasm, a man may be having a retrograde ejaculation—he is going instead of coming, so to speak.

Every year thousands of men have the operation, and of course many of them like to talk about it. A man contemplating such an operation could profit by talking with those who have had it.

WHAT TO DO BEFORE YOU SEE YOUR PHYSICIAN AND UROLOGIST

"Be prepared," the Boy Scouts once taught many of us. It's a lesson we could do well to follow today visiting the doctor. Get information—about your symptoms and circumstances, your family history, and your medical records. Whether this is gained via informational Internet sites or from your own research, certain things should be done prior to seeing your physician to make your visit more productive. A physician's time is very limited and if you have your information readily available, you can ask the proper questions and get the right answers.

Every man over fifty years of age (over forty if you have a history of prostate cancer in your family tree) should see a physician yearly and have an examination for their private parts. Things to be checked:

- *PSA* Make sure there has been no ejaculation or other manipulation of the prostate three days prior to any PSA blood test. That means no intercourse, masturbation, or even bike riding. Also make sure you have no symptoms of burning, abnormally frequent urination, fever, or chills prior to the PSA test.
- *Symptom score* Take the International or American Urologic Association test, seen in chapter 12. Go to the doctor armed with your score. Also check the PSA value relative to your age group in the tables.
- *Flow* When you go to void, have a full bladder; check your flow by urinating into a graduated receptacle. A kitchen

79

household cup is adequate if you know the graduations; 30 cubic centiliters (cc's) per ounce is the usual size. Flow for ten seconds and collect the flow, then calculate your flow per second: 100 cc's flow in 10 seconds, for example, is equal to 10 ccs per second—borderline low flow. Do this at least three or four times and take this information to your physician and urologist. Incidentally, many patients say that their urinary flow is better after ejaculating, and better flow is noted after ejaculation for a day or two in elderly men with benign prostatic hypertrophy (BPH).

A visit to the physician can yield any number of findings, two being benign prostatic hyperplasia (see page 64) and cancer (see page 69). Should the former be revealed, discuss the treatments available and the merits of starting with a trial of medication such as an alpha blocker like Cardura, Hyrtin, or Flomax. Ask too about alternative medications and other less invasive treatments, but do not avoid asking about the standard old treatment of transurethral resection.

If carcinoma of the prostate is found, ask your physician about radical prostatectomy, both retropubic or perineal types with and without pelvic lymph-node resection. Also ask about laparoscopic prostatectomy, a procedure developed in France in the last few years now done at a few centers in the United States. It is highly technical and not for everyone— patients and medical professionals alike—but it is highly effective when done by a urologist with expertise in laparoscopic surgery. Radiation therapy is also an option, with conformal external bean and/or seed therapy being the most commonly pursued.

AVOIDING THE KNIFE

In virtually any circumstance, every man hopes to avoid the knife. When it comes to the prostate, new techniques may correct your problem and obviate the need for surgery. Often, watchful waiting on symptoms is recommended, because in some patients prostate-obstructive symptoms tend to level off to an acceptable level after some time. When treatment is undertaken, it is my opinion that drug therapy should be the first choice. In the past decade, alpha-blockers terazosin, doxazosin, and tamsulosin (respectively marketed as Hyrtin, Cardura, and Flomax) have been prescribed to relax the prostate and bladder-neck muscles by acting on the nerves in these areas and thereby improving urine flow. Another drug, finasteride (Proscar) blocks a testosterone-like chemical. Taken once per day, this medication—like the others, administered orally—can shrink the prostate in some men, and thus reduce their urinary symptoms.

In addition to drug therapy, there are a number of treatments that vary in degree of invasiveness. Urologists use these latter treatments when drug therapy is ineffective. Transurethral microwave therapy uses heat to damage prostate tissue and a cooling system to protect the urethra from damage. While it does not cure BPH, microwave therapy does, however, help alleviate urinary frequency, urgency, straining, and intermittent flow. Another technique, transurethral needle ablation, uses low-level radio frequency, energy delivered through needles, to heat the prostate. It too seeks to shield the urethra from damage. Neither microwave therapy nor needle ablation, nor the medications, appears to affect

Procedure	Description
Radical Prostatectomy	Surgically removes the prostate and surrounding tissue. Recommended when cancer has not spread outside the prostate gland or is contained within the prostate gland.
External-Beam Radiation	X rays are focused on cancer area; used when cancer is still confined to the prostate gland or to reduce the size of the tumor. Conformal computerized localization is used now to further delineate the tumor site and increase the targeted radiation dose.
Brachytherapy	For tumors that haven't spread yet, small radioactive seeds are implanted in the prostate, where they give off cancer-killing radiation over a period of weeks or months. Different types of seeds are employed for the different treatment techniques available.
Hormone Therapy	Hormonal supplements and other drugs are used to reduce testosterone, which can cause prostate cancer cells to grow. Most often used when cancers have spread to areas outside the prostate or recurred.
Chemotherapy	Anticancer drugs are an option for patients when disease is widespread or has not responded to hormone treatment.

potency or cause incontinence in the vast majority of patients.

Other treatments being tried include balloon dilitation of the prostatic urethra, which has not yielded favorable results and thus is rarely used, and stents, early use of which was initially considered favorable, only to see long-term results not up to the standards of other techniques.

RADICAL PROSTATECTOMY

Other than skin cancer, prostate cancer is the most commonly diagnosed cancer among men in the United States. Only lung cancer takes more lives. Although we don't know the natural history of this disease or how to prevent it, it seems to be very treatable when detected early.

Prostate cancer usually has no symptoms in its early stages, so the only chance one has for early detection is a PSA test and digital rectal examination during an annual checkup. If your father or brother has had prostate cancer, you are at risk, so starting at age forty you should be checked yearly.

When symptoms do appear, they can be similar to those of an enlarged but noncancerous prostate: various problems with urination. But a doctor may also find a hard spot, bump, or asymmetry on the side of the prostate during his routine digital rectal examination, and that is a strong indication of cancer. The only sure way to diagnose this insidious cancer, however, is to take samples of the prostate gland with a needle under ultrasound guidance.

If cancer is diagnosed, it is mandatory that the physician determine the extent of the cancerous growth. The PSA blood test and bone scans will help determine the extent of the cancer. If the cancer is quite active microscopically from the biopsy, say a Gleason grade 8 on a scale of 10, an operation would not be recommended. Similarly, when cancer has spread beyond the prostate, no operation can cure it.

Prostate cancer generally progresses slowly, so some men opt when diagnosed for a "watchful waiting" treatment program. Other treatments include surgery—such as a radical prostatectomy—radiation therapy, hormone therapy, and chemotherapy. These therapies can be used alone or in combination, depending on the clinical circumstances; the stage and aggressiveness of the tumor determine the methods to be used in any cancer treatment. Among other side effects, impotence and incontinence can result from some treatment methods, and thorough discussion of these factors should be undertaken before any treatment is selected.

If the transurethral prostate resection is a minor tune-up, a radical prostatectomy is a major repair. In contrast to the resection, which chips away obstructing tissue, the radical prostatectomy is the complete removal of the prostate, as well as the pouch-like seminal vesicles behind it. Because both the gland and the vesicles produce the seminal fluid that carries sperm to and through the penis, their removal means that a man who has undergone a radical prostatectomy can no longer father children. Hence, younger men undergoing this procedure should consider freezing their sperm for future use and discuss this option with their physicians.

There are three types of radical prostatectomy: retropubic, standard, and laparoscopic. A radical retropubic prostatectomy removes the prostate and surrounding tissue via an abdominal incision; pelvic lymph nodes may be removed as well. A perineal prostatectomy is less invasive, removing the prostate through an opening between the scrotum and anus. In this case, if lymph nodes are to be removed, that surgery is done through a separate incision in the abdomen.

Prostate surgery removes nerve and blood vessels on the back of the prostate and can damage tissues surrounding the prostate area, with the result often being incontinence and impotence. Some men, for reasons that are poorly understood, simply remain potent despite the removal of these nerves and blood vessels that are felt to be very important in erectile function.

In an attempt to lessen the risk of postoperative impotence, some surgeons attempt a so-called nerve-sparing surgery. In the nerve-sparing operation, special care is taken to avoid harming the nerves and blood vessels that run through the back side of the prostate. In successful nerve-sparing surgeries, urinary incontinence and impotence are less likely to result after prostatectomy. Where this is not used or fails, special nerve grafts have been used in some instances to restore erections or maintain them after radical prostate surgery.

So why aren't all procedures the nerve-sparing variety? Because some urologists feel that this lack of complete removal of the prostate increases the chance that some cancer cells will be left behind with those nerves.

Who's right? Only time will tell for sure as we follow these men for decades after their nerve-sparing surgery to see if they have a higher rate of recurrence or not. It is a very good idea to discuss with your urologist the options and what his preference for surgery is before surgery is scheduled.

Whatever the case in that particular matter, surgery for prostate cancer has undergone significant refinements, and complication rates have been reduced dramatically over the past decade. The ten-year disease-specific survival after prostatectomy rate is more than 90 percent at this time, with less than 5 percent of patients developing bothersome urinary incontinence. Moreover, Viagra (sildenafil citrate) has helped patients with regard to postoperative sexual function. The need for blood transfusions has decreased significantly and hospital stay is usually limited to two or three days.

On the surgical-procedure front, laparoscopic radical prostatectomy has gained favor in France, with good early clinical results on patient survival. A subspeciality of urologic surgery, the laparoscopic radical prostatectomy is a difficult operation but when the technique becomes more widespread and is adopted by American urologists, it may become the treatment of choice for otherwise healthy patients with a localized prostate cancer.

After radical prostatectomy, leaking is not uncommon, nor is impotence. The incidence of these two complications of radical prostatectomy varies among surgeons who report their series in the literature of the field. By and large, incontinence ranges from 2 to 30 percent, depending on the surgeon, and impotence occurs in 10 to 60 percent of cases, again depending on the surgeon and whether nerve-sparing surgery was possible or attempted. Age, too, is a big factor in impotence following radical prostatectomy. In general, men below sixty years of age who undergo nerve-sparing surgery do better than older men.

It is best to wait a year after your radical surgery before you decide that you are indeed incontinent, totally or partially. Although most men will experience some minimal leakage or incontinence following prostate removal, most are "dry" again within a year. When incontinence is present, there are two basic varieties of the problem: total incontinence, where no control over urine flow or in-between voiding is possible, and stress incontinence, in which you lose a little control only under certain conditions such as coughing or sneezing. Stress incontinence is much more likely to be temporary, and the first remedy for it is to start doing Kegel exercises.

I prefer to call Kegels "winks," because to do them you kind of "wink" a contraction of your pelvic-floor muscles. I recommend a series of twenty to twenty-five "winks" three times per day. It is essential to perform this exercise every day to regain and maintain control of your urinary function after radical surgery. This little exercise has helped many people gain better bladder control and enabled them to control their urinary flow to a reasonable, tolerable level. Still, some may wish to wear a pad for insurance so that they don't stain light-colored trousers. For others, there is always the old penile clamp, which wraps around the penis and urethra and can be used in the totally incontinent patient.

For a small number of men, control never will come back, and in such patients, surgery may be necessary to correct the condition. The most common procedure is implantation of what is known as an "artificial sphincter," which takes the place of the muscles you used to use to control your urination. In this operation, a urologist surgically implants a cuff around the urethra and places the control valve in your scrotum. The cuff squeezes your urethra closed; to urinate, you simply squeeze the control in your scrotum. When you let the control go, the cuff squeezes shut and there is neither drip nor dribble in most patients. The other alternative, of course, is absorbent undergarments for adults. These are particularly useful when the problem is not severe. You can try a few different brands to see which one is most comfortable and suitable for your problem.

RADIATION THERAPY

Radiation therapy uses high-energy rays to stop cancer cells from growing. This treatment can be used in early-stage prostate cancer or after surgery to destroy any cancer cells that might remain after removal of the prostate. Whether cancer remains is determined by the pathologic examination of the specimen removed and careful examination of all the edges of the prostate. Radiation therapy may also be used for pain relief in advanced stages of prostate cancer that have spread to the bone.

There are two types of radiation therapy: external-beam and internal radiation, or brachytherapy. With external beam radiation, a machine beams X rays directly at the prostate from outside the body. Today, the technique involves a very accurate procedure called 3-D conformal radiation therapy, in which a computer target is used to determine the exact area of the cancer and the configuration of the prostate very precisely and limit damage to surrounding tissue areas. In brachytherapy, radioactive seeds are implanted into the prostate through an incision in the perineal area. They are placed in a grid fashion in order to equally irradiate all areas of the prostate.

Radiation therapy for prostate cancer has changed dramatically in the last thirty years. Radiation therapists have come to the conclusion that radiation doses used in the 1970s and 1980s may have been inadequate for optimal control of prostate cancer. New techniques have focused on improved dose delivery to the prostate with minimal exposure to the surrounding normal tissue. Three-dimensional conformal radiation therapy is the technique of choice at the present time.

Side effects of radiation therapy vary from none to fatigue, diarrhea, frequent and uncomfortable urination, and impotence. Impotence is less likely to occur with brachytherapy, but men also experience some rectal pain when this method is used.

HORMONE THERAPY

Prostate cancer is fed by testosterone. Removal of the testicles, or orchiectomy, is by far the simplest and most radical way to shut off testosterone production. Most men, however, do not like the idea of giving up their testicles, so hormone therapy is another treatment option for prostate cancer. There are several types of hormone therapy, which seeks to reduce the level of male hormones in the body. Luteinizing hormone-release hormone (LHRH) antagonists, for instance, prevent the testicles from producing testosterone. In the past, the female hormone estrogen has been given in the form of DES (diethylstilbestrol), because this hormone also counteracts testosterone.

While these treatments prevent production of testosterone in the testicles, some male hormones are still produced by the adrenal glands. In cases where this is a problem, a drug that blocks the effect of any remaining male hormones—an antiandrogen—is administered. Estrogen is one of these, but past studies of estrogen given to men with a history of heart disease has shown it can cause difficulties, thus it is not recommended. Other hormones have worked better and hormone therapy can keep cancer controlled for years. Furthermore, it has been very successful in relieving symptoms and pain in selected patients.

CHEMOTHERAPY

Chemotherapy, either given intravenously or taken orally, has been used to control pain and growth of cancer of the prostate.

GENE THERAPY

The goal of gene therapy for prostate cancer is to introduce genetic material into the malignant cell in an attempt to bring about either restoration of normal cellular function or, more commonly, tumor-cell death. Many clinical trials along various lines of therapy are now in progress. Watch your newspapers for the latest therapy or ask your urologist if there is anything new along the genome trail.

CHAPTER EIGHT

SEXUALLY TRANSMITTED DISEASES

Once, they were called venereal diseases, but they now have a new name: sexually transmitted diseases. Some of their number, such as syphilis and gonorrhea, linger but have receded from past prominence, while newcomers, like AIDS, present unprecedented and alarming challenges and other old stand-bys, herpes and hepatitis B among them, have caught popular attention anew. But whoever today's stars are and whether they're called VD or STDs, they're here to stay.

Listed below are America's most troublesome sexually transmitted diseases.

SYPHILIS

Syphilis (syph, gumma) has been around a very long time. It swept across Europe in the latter part of the fifteenth century; some historians believe that it was brought from North America by members of Columbus's crew or that of another explorer of the time, while others think the opposite occurred. Whatever the case, syphilis has been known to be in America since the continent was discovered by Europeans.

Syphilis can be effectively cured if treated immediately with penicillin. If it goes untreated, though, and is allowed to reach its advanced stage—years after infection—it can cause paralysis, insanity, blindness, and even death. The bacteria that cause syphilis, spiral-shaped microorganisms called *Treponema pallidum,* are transmitted by sexual contact, by touching an infected sore, or by direct contact with infected blood. They also can be transferred from a pregnant woman to her fetus.

If allowed to run its course, syphilis occurs in three stages:

Primary   The first indication of syphilis is a chancre (pronounced SHANK-er) which appears about two to four weeks after infection. It begins as a dull red spot, then becomes a pimple, then ulcerates into a round or oval sore with a crater-like edge. This is the chancre. The sore is roughly the color of raw ham, is firm, and is neither tender nor painful. Even if untreated, it usually heals in three or four weeks, leaving the impression that the problem has gone away. This is part of syphilis's deception.

Secondary   If the syphilis has been treated with penicillin in its early stage, no doubt it will be cured. But if not, a second stage will follow at some time between a week and six months after the chancre has healed. Symptoms of the second stage include a pale or pinkish rash on the palms of the hands and soles of the feet, fever, a sore throat, headaches, pains in the joints, hair loss, a poor appetite, and even weight loss. The most serious symptoms, though, are open sores that appear on the genitals and anus and are highly contagious. Because of its variety of symptoms and signs that are also characteristic of other diseases, syphilis is sometimes called the great imitator and is often diagnosed incorrectly. This is another aspect of its deception.

This second stage usually lasts three to six months, although it can recur periodically. Then, all symptoms disappear and the syphilis seems to have gone away again. Instead, however, it has entered another dormant period. It is no longer contagious, but its infections enter and grow in other parts of the body.

Tertiary This is late syphilis, and usually shows up years after the first stage. It is marked by serious problems with the brain, spinal cord, eyes, heart, or wherever the infections have been growing. Severe complications can cause insanity, paralysis, blindness, and even death.

GONORRHEA

Gonorrhea (the clap, the drip) is the oldest known sexually transmitted disease. Moses himself was instructed to warn of its uncleanness in the Old Testament (Leviticus 15), and Plato, Aristotle, and Hippocrates all mentioned it. It is one of the most common infectious diseases. In the United States alone, more than a million cases are reported each year, though the actual number of new cases may be many times that.

Gonorrhea has a short incubation period, with symptoms—primary among them is a yellowish discharge from the penis—appearing anywhere from one to eight days after infection. The transmission route is through sexual contact, be it intercourse, fellatio, or anal intercourse. In addition, there is evidence that inanimate objects may also spread gonorrhea—which means that that old "I caught it on a toilet seat" excuse is not as lame as it seems. My own experiments showed that the gonorrhea bacteria in their natural state last as long as two hours on a toilet seat or wet toilet paper. And although this route of asexual transmission is rare, it is at least theoretically possible, as described in the *New England Journal of Medicine* in 1979.*

New strains of gonoccocal organisms may resist penicillin, the old standard treatment. Penicillin and Erythromycin should not be used in the United States of America for treatment of gonorrhea today. Use current treatment guidelines of the CDC published by the Centers for Disease Prevention and Control, available by calling (800) 342-AIDS (2437).

VENEREAL WARTS

Venereal warts are growths that occur in cool, moist areas, particularly around the penis, scrotum, and anus. They have a white, rough surface, something like a cauliflower, and grow singly or in clusters. They are painless and can be easily removed, for although benign, their ugly appearance could deter a potential sex partner. Warts may coexist with other sexually transmitted diseases, and are probably the most contagious of them all. The virus is passed by sexual contact and survives well outside the body.

---

* For more details, see "The Gonococcus and the Toilets Seat," *New England Journal of Medicine* 301 (July 12, 1979): 91–93.

GENITAL HERPES

Genital herpes is a virally transmitted skin infection that affects some 20 million people, many of whom carry it for life because there is no known cure. Some individuals may have only one outbreak in a lifetime, but others may have many, often instigated by stress or depression. The signs of an outbreak are the appearance of small pimples that burn with pain. Some blisters appear singly, but most develop in clusters of ten to twenty on the penis, urethra, or rectum in men, and on the vaginal lips, cervix, or rectum in women. A tingling sensation may precede the pimples, and the first outbreak may be accompanied by a fever, headache, burning urination, discharge from the penis, and swollen glands in the groin.

After a few days the headache and fever will fade away and the pimples will burst and form open sores. The sores will crust over and heal in about two weeks, leaving the patient with the impression that the herpes has gone. Instead, the herpes virus will have moved into a dormant stage and, in 90 percent of cases, will strike again. The time of the next attack and the pattern of subsequent attacks vary from a few weeks to many years. Recurrent attacks may be stimulated by emotional distress, physical exhaustion, illness, sunburn, or maybe for no evident reason at all. Subsequent attacks are likely to be less severe because the body is prepared for them, and their timing may vary considerably, but herpes almost always comes back.

CRABS

A very common affliction, pubic lice (crabs) are small, white, oval-shaped bugs which under a microscope look like translucent ocean crabs. They are parasites that attach themselves to pubic hair and feed on blood obtained by biting their host.

Crab lice are transmitted during sexual contact, hair to hair. Although they are most prevalent in pubic hair, crabs can leap to eyebrows and eyelashes during fellatio or cunnilingus. They also can be acquired from sheets, towels, or clothing used by an infected person, for while the lice themselves can survive only twenty-four hours after they leave the human body, their eggs can survive up to six days in sheets or clothing. In such cases, a week will pass before crabs begin to itch. A newly acquired infection of live crabs, though, will be evident within a day. Although crabs are an irritant, infestation is not a serious disease. A few people even feel no symptoms, but most develop an itchy rash that can become infected.

An effective way to get rid of crabs is to apply a 1 percent gamma benzene hexachloride solution, which is available as a lotion or shampoo marketed under the trade name Kwell. Kwell lotion applied to pubic hair must be left on for twenty-four hours; Kwell shampoo should be rubbed into all hairy areas vigorously for ten minutes before being rinsed off. The shampoo treatment should be repeated in a week if any nits (crab eggs) remain. Eyelash infestation must be treated by applying petroleum ophthalmic ointment twice daily for ten days.

HEPATITIS B

Hepatitis B is one of many forms of viral hepatitis, a liver infection that can cause chills, fever, diarrhea, nausea, anorexia (the need to vomit), and possibly jaundice (a liver condition that turns the skin yellowish). Extreme consequences can be chronic liver disease and/or death.

Hepatitis B virus is transmitted through blood, saliva, seminal fluid, vaginal secretions, and other body fluids. Approximately 200,000 active cases are diagnosed annually in the United States, some of them sexually transmitted, but up to four times that many people may be hepatitis carriers—infected with the disease but not ill from it.

There is no known cure for hepatitis B, so the only treatment is supportive, or intended to make the patient feel better. A vaccine has been developed to act as a preventative, but it is not effective after the disease has been acquired.

MOLLUSCUM CONTAGIOSUM

Molluscum contagiosum is a painless skin lesion, a small pinkish or orange bump that, when squeezed, will pop a plug of material similar to a blackhead. It appears on the genitalia, thighs, buttocks, and lower abdomen. It does not cause much trouble and it often disappears, even without treatment, over a period of months.

CHANCROID

Chancroid is a sexually transmitted disease rare in the United States but common in the tropics. If your partner has been in a tropical climate, check with your doctor.

NONSPECIFIC URETHRITIS (NSU)

Nonspecific urethritis is an umbrella term for a category of relatively minor but rapidly spreading sexually transmitted diseases. Their common symptoms—discharge from the penis and pain while urinating—are also common to gonorrhea, but NSUs are not caused by the same organism. In fact, they resist treatment by penicillin, the usual cure for gonorrhea.

Chlamydia, one of the NSU group, is the most prevalent sexually transmitted disease in the United States. It is usually diagnosed by process of elimination—by determining what the patient's affliction is *not*. Tetracycline is usually an effective treatment. If chlamydia is left untreated, secondary infections can reach other organs and result in infertility.

The initials "NSU" seem more benign than the unambiguous *gonorrhea,* and for that reason NSU frequently appears in medical records. In the military, for example, officers and enlisted men will often go to town and do the same things, probably with the same women, and return to the base with the very same infections. But whereas the officers' records would note presence of some NSU, enlisted men's records would report infection by gonorrhea: the officers had the clout and the enlisted men had the clap.

ACQUIRED IMMUNE DEFICIENCY
SYNDROME (AIDS)

AIDS is caused by a human immunodeficiency virus (HIV), which is transmitted by sexual activity or by specific other means, such as transfusion of contaminated blood or use of contaminated drug paraphernalia. How AIDS is sexually transmitted—or not transmitted—is a subject of much misunderstanding. Perhaps this definition of transmission may help: Any sexual activity involving exposure to the blood, semen, or vaginal secretions of an HIV-infected person can result in AIDS-virus transmission.

AIDS was first reported in the United States in 1981, and there is good evidence that the number of cases is increasing each year. The disease breaks down the body's protective immune system, leaving it vulnerable to serious diseases, many of which are virtually unheard of when the immune system is functioning normally. The disease has reached epidemic status in the United States and worldwide. And although there is no known cure, the proper use of a condom and avoidance of certain sexual practices can reduce the risk of AIDS considerably.

In the face of such a serious threat, people ask the same questions over and over: How do I know if I don't have AIDS? How do I know that my sexual partners in the past ten to fifteen years did not have AIDS?

A first step toward answering these questions is to determine whether or not one or any of one's sexual partners belong to a high-risk group. Groups that have a high risk of acquiring AIDS include homosexual and bisexual men, intravenous-drug users, blood-transfusion recipients, and persons who have been sexually intimate with prostitutes or with members of the other high-risk groups. As the saying goes, you sleep with everyone your partner has slept with.

If a patient is truly concerned about the possibility of being HIV positive or developing AIDS, I recommend that he or she undergo a blood test, especially if he or she is in the high-risk category. A positive blood result indicates infection with HIV, but not necessarily AIDS itself. In fact, patients with full-blown AIDS may test negatively due to the inability of the body to make antibodies against the AIDS virus.

Positive tests will not occur right away, for antibodies to the AIDS virus will not appear in the blood for at least three weeks to six months after infection; sometimes it takes even longer. Medical science does not yet know how many years after exposure a person may still be at risk for a full-blown onset of AIDS. If you feel you want to be tested, see your physician or call the AIDS toll-free hotline at 1 (800) 342-AIDS (7514).

At this time in the United States, more physicians are becoming familiar with HIV infection and AIDS, but not all are sufficiently trained in this area. If your doctor is uncomfortable or unfamiliar with HIV or AIDS management, ask for a referral to an expert.

CHAPTER NINE

THE BLADDER

Nature arranged the various parts of a human urinary system from top to bottom to perform separate but related functions in a logical order.

At the top are the kidneys, which produce and process urine and pass it through tubes, called ureters, down into the bladder. Unlike other parts of the system, the bladder has only one function: it is a reservoir to hold and release urine. Its capacity is twelve to fifteen ounces, about equal in volume to a can of beer. Urine is held in the bladder until its release, when it exits the body via the urethra. As discussed in another chapter, in a man's body, the urethra passes through the prostate gland, which is immediately below the bladder neck, and through the penis to exit the body.

Because of their proximity, prostate and bladder functions are closely related, and problems of the prostate often become problems of the bladder. Obstructions or blockage of the prostate, for example, put pressure on bladder muscles, which must work harder to evacuate urine. The muscles begin to thicken and enlarge, just as biceps in the upper arm build up with heavy use. The thickening can reduce bladder capacity, requiring more frequent urination than normal. In other cases, pressure from the prostate may have an opposite effect and instead cause bladder muscles to stretch instead of thicken. This usually occurs after long-term blockage in the prostate. The distended bladder holds more urine than it should and does not empty completely with each voiding— only the top of the reservoir goes and most of the urine remains. The bladder is constantly almost full, and usually feels full.

Such was the circumstance of a seventy-year-old farmer who came in to see me—at the insistence of his wife—about his expanding girth. His wife, it seemed, had had to let out his pants to relieve pressure around his abdomen once too often, and she wanted to know why.

I asked him about his urinary habits. He said he spent long hours on his tractor and had trained himself to hold back his bladder so he wouldn't have to stop working to urinate. This had resulted in a greatly distended bladder. I drained off more than a quart of urine, which is more than twice the normal amount. I then performed a transurethral resection of his prostate to clear up a related problem. Now he is able to empty his bladder normally. He's wearing a smaller trouser size and he feels much more comfortable. Taking comfort to an even higher level, he gave the farm, along with his tractor, to his son, and drove his air-conditioned Cadillac to Palm Springs, where he and his wife bought a retirement condominium.

Stretching the bladder walls can also bring on diverticula, which are pouches or bubbles that distend from weak points on bladder walls. The bubbles, large or small, form when the bladder is under pressure, just as a weakened lining in an inner-tube wall swells disproportionately when the tube is inflated.

Another bladder condition, fortunately rare, is interstitial cystitis. It is characterized by low bladder capacity, bladder pain, and urination as frequent as three or four times an hour and five to ten times a night. The filling bladder often triggers severe pain, which can be relieved only by urination. The cause is not known, but close inspection in most cases reveals the existence of a bladder ulcer. More familiar bladder problems include inflammation, stones, and cancer. Inflammation of the bladder is often associated with inflammation of the prostate and usually can be treated with antibiotics. Stones are deposits of uric acid or calcium, something like deposits of scale in a radiator, and are caused by an obstruction of the prostate or mishandling of chemicals by the body. Stones can be passed naturally or be removed either mechanically or electrically.

The lining cells of the kidneys and the bladder, as well as of the ureter connecting them, all are of the same type. Cancer can develop in any of these, but the most common location is the bladder. Cigarette smoking, so often identified with lung cancer, also has been incriminated as a possible source of cancer of the bladder, because of a reaction between chemicals in cigarette smoke and lining cells in the urinary tract. A significant sign of cancer of the bladder is blood in the urine. It is painless bleeding, but it is a danger sign, as illustrated by the following case:

A chef, age forty-four, came in after experiencing painless urinary bleeding for three consecutive days. He had no prior history of bleeding, was otherwise relatively healthy, and his physical examination was normal, even though he was a two-pack-per-day smoker and had been for twenty-five years. X rays, however, showed normal kidneys but an abnormal mass in his bladder. The mass was malignant, and I removed it with a transurethral resection. The tumor was non-infiltrating, which meant that its roots were not so deeply embedded in the bladder as to prevent complete removal. Still, bladder tumors tend to recur, so close observation with regular follow-up was mandatory. He was also advised to quit smoking, which he did successfully.

Ruptures of the bladder or the urethra often occur in automobile accidents if the bladder is full. After an accident, trouble signs that mandate immediate attention are the presence of blood in the urine or no urine output—each can indicate damage to the bladder. Thus, as a precaution, anybody about to travel in a car should empty his bladder first. An empty bladder doesn't rupture, but a full bladder can burst like a ripe melon.

Any and all of these conditions may be investigated, diagnosed, and treated by a doctor using a couple of unique instruments. A cystoscope is a surgical instrument that resembles a miniature telescope, with a long extension for insertion up the penis through the urethra. With a water supply, to expand the bladder, and fiber-optic light source, it is capable of exploring the entire urinary tract—urethra, prostate, and bladder. With a smaller attachment, a doctor can also use the cytoscope to examine the kidneys for stones, tumors, or other abnormalities. A similar instrument, a resectoscope, has attachments for electric power and optics, and can remove bladder stones in several ways—mechanically, electrically, or ultrasonically. It can disintegrate stones from the size of peas to golf balls and flush out debris through the penis. No incision is required. Also, most bladder cancers can be removed with a resectoscope.

If cancerous tumors are found to be infiltrating the bladder wall, more drastic measures are necessary; an operation even may be required to remove the prostate and the bladder. In this extreme latter case, a segment of the small bowel is transplanted to serve as a reservoir, or a small bladder, joined directly to the kidneys, using ureters as urine conduits. Urine is drained from the substitute bladder into a small bag glued to the skin outside the body.

Incidentally, it should be known that certain foods can cause changes in the urine of some men. A distinct red tinge, for instance, may show up after eating beets. Often mistaken for blood, the color is due to the presence of betanin, a red pigment, not blood cells. Beeturia, though, is often misinterpreted as bloody urine by the unsuspecting. The pungent urinary odor produced by some individuals within a short time after eating asparagus can also be alarming. It is debatable whether the latter condition is a problem with how the body handles the chemistry in asparagus or is a sensitivity to the odor. These strange happenings are nothing to worry about.

To close on a light note, I offer this old story: A young man who had just entered Britain's diplomatic service was assigned to routine chores at an international conference where Winston Churchill was present. At one fortunate moment, the young man found himself alone with the great statesman.

Taking advantage of the opportunity, he asked Churchill for any advice appropriate for a young man entering His Majesty's diplomatic service.

Churchill pursed his lips for a moment, then replied, "Young man, never pass up the opportunity to take a leak."

CHAPTER TEN

THE HARD FACTS:
QUESTIONNAIRE RESULTS

Mike, a patient of mine, has a small garage where he has repaired all kinds of cars for all kinds of drivers during forty years in business. He has followed transmission trends from stick shifts to automatics and back to stick shifts; he has nursed hand throttles, automatic chokes, and fuel injectors.

And just as Mike has kept up with changes in cars, he has adjusted to changes in drivers. Some complain about the slightest squeak while others nurse the old buggy as long as it will stay on the road; some know absolutely nothing about a car, others volunteer diagnoses whether they're right or wrong.

Mike knows his customers and has concluded that drivers are like cars; all are similar, yet each is different. He might find outside validation for this in a survey I conducted to determine lifestyles and sex styles of one hundred men—in this case, business- and professional men who have achieved success in their thirty-five to fifty years of life. Many had advanced degrees, and all were affluent, with more than half earning at least $175,000 a year. Three-fourths of them were married and had two or three children. Ninety-six percent said they were heterosexual. Thirty-five percent had had vasectomies. Most claimed some church attendance (53 percent were Protestant, 21 percent Catholic, and 7 percent Jewish).

They were assured that the survey would be confidential and that their personal results would be disclosed only to them. With anonymity and with nobody looking over their shoulders, then, these gentlemen reported that they couldn't find much change in their sexual appetites and sexual prowess in the years since they were twenty-five, that they enjoyed and encouraged oral sex with their wives or girlfriends, and that intercourse was still the best way to go—though for some it now took longer.

Almost all of the men questioned were married or had been, and a third of those currently married admitted having sexual affairs. The number of extramarital partners ranged from one to an impressive, if incredible, ninety-eight. Apparently, they think marital fidelity is more essential for wives than for themselves, because 82 percent of the husbands thought their wives were faithful. Only one of these fellows acknowledged having lost all interest in sex; the others stayed keyed up. They rated appearance as the major attraction in the opposite sex, and the looks they were seeking out translated into breasts and buttocks—the formula that ignites fires in male imaginations. Here is what the study has revealed:

HEALTH

This was a healthy group. Most claimed health that was excellent or above average. Perhaps because they were feeling good, only one-third got annual physical examinations, some only because their companies or their wives required them to. Another third went to a doctor only when they were sick, and a few said going to a doctor didn't do any good.

None had had a heart attack, two-thirds exercised with some regularity—some vigorously, some languidly—and more than half said they maintained a healthy diet, had cut down on consumption of red meat, and had reduced salt intake in the past few years.

Some (13 percent) had high blood pressure, a possible cause of impotence, but only 4 percent took medication for hypertension. One in four reported a family history of diabetes, and two-thirds said the health problem they feared most was cancer.

Drinking was out completely for three of every ten respondents. More (60 percent) drank two to four ounces a day, whether hard liquor, wine, or beer, and 10 percent drank more than four ounces a day. Only one in ten said he drank alcohol at a business lunch.

Most (88 percent) did not smoke cigarettes.

Perhaps because they enjoyed good health, very few acknowledged being too tired to do things.

In employment, almost all enjoyed positions with authority and were satisfied with their careers, and every single one (100 percent) felt good about his future.

MARRIAGE

Just 5 percent of these men were single. The others were in various stages of matrimony: married (78 percent), divorced

(15 percent), or separated (2 percent). Of those who were married, 72 percent had married once, 23 percent twice, and 5 percent three or more times. Most had two or three children.

Most husbands judged that their lives with their wives were pleasurable (44 percent) or very pleasurable (44 percent). When asked in more specific terms, they offered these results, still generally favorable: Half reported a central satisfaction with life lived with their mates, and 19 percent said they vitally shared everything with their wives. But 12 percent conceded conflict or controlled tension (albeit discreet and polite), 9 percent admitted that marriage had dulled in middle age, and 7 percent acknowledged boring and routine marriages with emphasis on other things.

Every husband said communication with his wife was important. The subjects most frequently mentioned were money, children, and use of leisure time. About eight men in ten said that they were comfortable discussing sex with their wives, and that conversation often starts in the kitchen. Each executive was asked to identify his best friend, and more than half named their wives. More than a third would go first to their wives for personal advice (best friends were second, chosen by 22 percent). One man in five had considered divorce; usually he was deterred because of the children. Fewer than half (41 percent) of married men wore wedding rings.

EXTRAMARITAL AFFAIRS

One-third of these husbands acknowledged having had an affair. Specifically, 34 percent admitted having extramarital intercourse, 61 percent denied it, and 4 percent said it wasn't applicable, whatever that means. One bachelor said he was having an affair, presumably cheating on his girlfriend.

Some (17 percent) said they had patronized prostitutes in the previous five years.

Answers to the fidelity question varied according to the respondent's number of marriages. Each was asked to respond to this question regarding his present marital relationship. Among once-married men, 40 percent acknowledged affairs; among twice-married, 22 percent, and among the few married three or more times, two-thirds admitted having had affairs. Evidently these fellows had given up on marriage as an institution.

Asked how many other women they had had during their marriages, most husbands ranged between one and five. About 20 percent said one only, but one prodigious fellow claimed to have slept with ninety-eight women. Most of these fellows liked extracurricular affairs; 85 percent rated them pleasurable or very pleasurable.

Were wives playing the same game? Presumably not: Only 10 percent of the husbands knew their wives were cheating, or thought they were, and 82 percent trusted their wives. Did the women know about their men? The conjecture among husbands was split, 50–50.

PERFORMANCE

Most men said they had sexual intercourse from one to four times a week; one-third said twice a week. Only 4 percent reported no sex at all during a week.

When does all this happen? It appears that ten o'clock on Saturday night is a poor time to call the boss. Saturday night is still the action night, cited by 43 percent of respondents, and ten o'clock is happy hour—a choice of 45 percent. Other preferred days were Sundays and Fridays; the second favored hour was the next morning.

Who does the arousing? Men get things started, or think they do, on about two-thirds of all occasions; men and women initiate sex together the other third of the time. But very seldom does a wife initiate sex herself. This arrangement seemed satisfactory to only about 60 percent of those surveyed; the rest said things might be better if wives initiated sex more frequently.

Nearly all men surveyed (92 percent) had performed cunnilingus and most (85 percent) enjoyed it. Three-fourths of the men enjoyed fellatio, but only half of them thought their wives liked it too. Oral sex often served as a preliminary to intercourse.

Once intercourse began, a substantial majority of the men (93 percent) said they achieved orgasm every time or almost every time. The rest claimed orgasm about three-fourths of the time. About one-fourth of them (23 percent) said they thought their mates climaxed three-quarters of the time; twice as many men (46 percent) surmised that their partners reached orgasm half the time. Half the men claimed they could climax in two to five minutes; a very few (2 percent) said they had to work fifteen minutes to half an hour. Most (88 percent) had only one orgasm a night, but 10 percent said they could come twice, and a very few (2 percent) asserted they could come three times.

Some men conceded that it didn't always come out the way they'd have liked. More than half (59 percent) admitted they had failed to achieve or maintain an erection at some point. The causes, in order cited, were being too tired, having too much to drink, or being with a new partner for the first time. A few men (18 percent) admitted having a different problem: premature ejaculation. And, surprisingly, 15 percent said they had faked orgasm at one time or another.

Men think and dream about sex. Eighty-four percent of those surveyed do, at least. But our respondents reported that nocturnal erections and wet dreams became rarer as they grew older, and half of them said they didn't have wet dreams anymore.

LOST YOUTH

If these fellows answered their questions accurately, they hadn't lost a whole lot from their sexual prime back when they were twenty-five years old. By almost two to one, they claimed it didn't take them any longer to get an erection now than it had at age twenty-five, that they didn't require any more penile stroking to reach orgasm than in those heydays, and that the volume of ejaculate spurting from those erections was as much as it ever was. By three to one, they claimed their penises got as stiff as before and stayed stiff during sex. The big admitted loss, from those days of youth, was rejuvenation—three-fourths conceded it did take longer to get another erection after orgasm than it once had.

Practically every respondent said that he was easily or very easily aroused sexually, just as he had been at age twenty-five. Half said sex was more enjoyable. The opposite was true for masturbation, for 75 percent said they masturbated less frequently than they had at age eighteen—although 6 percent said they masturbated more.

Almost all men (95 percent) claimed their erections were as big as they ever were, and that they rose without pain. A few noticed that their penises would bend, and a few more (11 percent) said they had ejaculated without erections. As a matter of fact, both occurrences are normal.

Not that anything could be done about it, but each respondent was asked, just for fun, if he'd like to have a larger, more formidable penis. Given this choice, one-third of them said they'd like their erections another inch longer, please, and one in four would prefer another inch in circumference. Perhaps it is more significant that all of the others were satisfied with their present dimensions. Maybe that was because only 18 percent of the men thought their wives or girlfriends would welcome a larger erection, and only 18 percent hoped to encounter a tighter vagina.

Something can be done about creating erections artificially (as described earlier, surgical implantation of penile prostheses can remedy the situation) if natural erection fails. Half the men questioned said they would favorably consider such an operation if matters came (or didn't come) to that. These answers indicate that acceptance of artificial devices has increased significantly in the last several years.

A few questions near the end of the lengthy survey, reached after the responding executives had put a good deal of time and thought into their answers, disclosed how much these fellows really were interested in sex.

Dominating answers to a multiple-choice question about ways to improve sex life were appeals for more: more frequent intercourse (64 percent), the partner should initiate sex more often (40 percent), more frequent oral sex (46 percent), and more spontaneous sex (40 percent).

Finally, the men were given a chance to get away from it all by checking off their favorite extracurricular activities. Sex was the second most popular activity, named by 16 percent of the respondents. Leading the list, the choice of 22 percent, was golf.

CHAPTER ELEVEN

PERSONAL EQ:
ERECTILE QUOTIENT QUIZ

The following is a personal inventory of sexual impotence risks.

Answer questions 1–15 by circling YES or NO in the column on the right.

1. I have sugar diabetes.   YES   NO
2. I have high blood pressure (hypertension).   YES   NO
3. I take medication for high blood pressure.   YES   NO
4. I smoke cigarettes.   YES   NO
5. I take medication for heart irregularity.   YES   NO
6. I find that I am often too tired to do anything,
   and the future seems hopeless.   YES   NO
7. My present weight is more than ten pounds
   over my ideal weight.*   YES   NO
8. I am happy with my career choice.   YES   NO
9. I am satisfied with my mate.   YES   NO
10. My daily diet is best described as balanced.   YES   NO

* "Ideal weight" is the weight determined by actuarial tables to be healthy for one's height and age.

11. In the last few years, I have decreased red-meat consumption in my diet.   YES   NO

12. I am satisfied with my sexual variety.   YES   NO

13. My erection has shown no change compared to my earlier years.   YES   NO

14. My erection has shown some change compared to my earlier years.   YES   NO

15. My penis is as firm and hard as it was in the past.   YES   NO

Choose the most appropriate response for questions 16–20.

16. I drink alcohol in this amount:
    a. more than two ounces per day
    b. up to two ounces per day
    c. none

17. My exercise program is best described as:
    a. none
    b. mild or regular
    c. vigorous

18. I need more stimulation to get an erection now than I did in earlier years:
    a. big change
    b. some change
    c. no change

19. After ejaculation, it takes me longer to get another erection now than it did in earlier years:
    a. yes
    b. some change
    c. no change

20. My interest in sex now, compared to my interest in it in earlier years, is:
    a. less strong
    b. same
    c. stronger

KEY TO PERSONAL EQ

Questions 1–7: 0 points for each YES; 10 points for each NO.
Questions 8–15: 10 points for each YES; 0 points for each NO.
Questions 16–20: Give yourself 0 points for each "a" response, 5 points for each "b," and 10 points for each "c."

Add up your total points. The average score is 125. If your score is 100 or below, consult your doctor.

CHAPTER TWELVE

Personal Inventory of Your Bladder Habits

If you are approaching fifty years of age, don't feel embarrassed to talk to your doctor about urinary problems. These two quizzes are designed to give a short test to measure the severity of urinary symptoms and assign a number to it. These numbers may change over the years. The maximum possible score is 35. The final question will help you judge how your feel about your symptoms. This test was designed and compiled by a number of urologists in the United States and around the world to try to get a handle on the severity of your symptoms and merely produces a number. It is not a diagnostic test to determine whether you have benign prostatic hyperplasia. To know even if you have reason for concern, you must take this test several times and talk with your doctor regarding your symptoms. This test score is not intended to substitute for medical treatment.

Remember: Don't be embarrassed to talk about your symptoms, getting up at night, slow stream, dribbling, double voiding, and the like. It is a very common problem everywhere. By the age of fifty, one in four males will require treatment for their urinary symptoms caused by benign prostatic hyperplasia. Take the quiz and you and your doctor can decide if you could benefit from some type of treatment.

Approximately 50 percent of men over the age of fifty have demonstrated benign prostatic hyperplasia. Only one in five men will require some form of operation for the treatment of their symptoms. In this day and age of newer medications, medical management for discomfort and irritation related to benign prostatic hyperplasia is in order and should be the first line of treatment. A careful history by your physician or urologist is mandatory to determine which treatment or if any treatment is necessary.

The American Urological Association has developed some practice guidelines, which is an easy test for patients to take and score themselves. You can check the severity of your own symptoms. This score, along with a careful history and physical examination that includes a digital rectal examination of your prostate, should be undertaken before any treatment is started. The symptom score should be used by all physicians treating men with benign prostatic hyperplasia. The big problems of urinary tract infection, recurrent gross blood in your urine, bladder stones, and obstructive symptoms as demonstrated by bladder and renal dysfunction should all be checked out. Most patients with bladder obstruction symptoms and irritability will do best with a trial medication.

It is a good idea for all men after fifty years (or before, if symptoms persist) to take this simple test and find out what their grade is. Patients with mild symptoms—a score of less than 7—could possibly just wait and watch and see if symptoms get worse. The moderate symptoms, 8–19 on this test, should see their urologist and discuss the symptoms with him or her. Severe symptoms—over 20 on this test—are indicative of serious obstruction, and urologic consultation should be in order. Your urologist will decide on your treatment. It is a good idea to take this test several times, write the numbers down and discuss it with your urologist.

American Urological Association and International Prostate Symptom Score (I-PSS) Quiz

You may feel embarrassed to talk to your doctor about urinary problems. But, like gray and thinning hair, such problems are a part of aging. One of the causes of urinary symptoms in men over fifty is a treatable condition called benign prostatic hyperplasia (BPH). In fact, it has been estimated that by the age of eighty, one in every four males in the U.S. will require treatment of their urinary symptoms caused by BPH.*

Take this quiz to help you and your doctor decide whether you could benefit from a BPH treatment.

TAKING THE QUIZ
Please circle the answer that best represents your response to each of the following questions. The questions are designed to gauge the severity of any symptoms you may be experiencing.

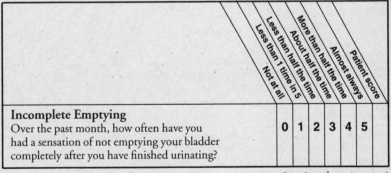

	Not at all	Less than 1 time in 5	Less than half the time	About half the time	More than half the time	Almost always	Patient score
Incomplete Emptying Over the past month, how often have you had a sensation of not emptying your bladder completely after you have finished urinating?	0	1	2	3	4	5	

(continued on next page)

* McConnell, J. D., Barry, M. J., Bruskewitz, R. C., et al. *Benign Prostatic Hyperplasia: Diagnosis and Treatment.* Clinical Practice Guideline, Number 8. AHCPR Publication No. 94-0582. Rockville, Md: Agency for Health Care Policy and Research, Public Health Service, U.S. Department of Health and Human Services. February 1994.

Frequency Over the past month, how often have you had to urinate again less than two hours after you have finished urinating?	0 1 2 3 4 5
Intermittency Over the past month, how often have you found you stopped and started again several times when you urinated?	0 1 2 3 4 5
Urgency Over the past month, how often have you found it difficult to postpone urination?	0 1 2 3 4 5
Weak Stream Over the past month, how often have you had a weak urinary stream?	0 1 2 3 4 5
Straining Over the past month, how often have you had to push or strain to begin urination?	0 1 2 3 4 5
Nocturia Over the past month, how many times did you most typically get up to urinate from the time you went to bed at night until the time you got up in the morning?	0 1 2 3 4 5+
	Your Total Score

	Delighted	Pleased	Mostly satisfied	Mixed	Mostly dissatisfied	Unhappy	Terrible
Quality of Life Due to Urinary Symptoms If you were to spend the rest of your life with your urinary condition the way it is now, how would you feel about that?	0	1	2	3	4	5	6

Adapted from Barry, M. J., et al. The American Urological Association symptom index for benign prostatic hyperplasia. *Journal of Urology* 1992;148:1549–57.

SCORING THE QUIZ
Add the numbers from your answers to questions 1 through 7. The maximum possible score is 35. The final question will help you judge how you feel about your symptoms.

PLEASE NOTE: This test is used to measure the severity of your symptoms. It is not a diagnostic test. In other words, it will not tell you whether or not you have BPH. Talk to your doctor to determine whether your symptoms are due to BPH.

Remember: This information is not intended as a substitute for medical treatment.

SCORING THE QUIZ

The International Prostate Symptoms Score (I-PSS) is based on the answers to seven questions concerning urinary symptoms. Each question allows the patient to choose one of five answers indicating increasing severity of the particular symptom. The answers are assigned points from 0 to 5. The total score can therefore range from 0 to 35 (asymptomatic to very symptomatic). Furthermore, the International Consensus Committee (ICC) recommends the use of only a single question to assess the quality of life. The answers to this question range from "delighted" to "terrible," or 0 to 6. Although this single question may or may not capture the global impact of BPH symptoms or quality of life, it may serve as a valuable starting point for a doctor-patient conversation. The ICC strongly recommends that all physicians who counsel patients suffering from symptoms of prostatism utilize these measures not only during the initial interview but also during and after treatment in order to monitor treatment response.*

FLOW RATE

Another way to define problems with benign prostatic hyperplasia is to test your flow. Electronic equipment is available for flow rate, but there is a simpler way to check your flow pe-

---

* The ICC under the patronage of the World Health Organization (WHO) has agreed to use the symptom index for benign prostatic hypertrophy (BPH), which has been developed by the American Urological Association (AUA) Measurement Committee, as the official worldwide symptoms-assessment tool for patients.

riodically at home by yourself and also let your urologist know. More complex problems are usually investigated with fancy urodynamic studies including video and other electronic studies.

Here is a way you can check your own urine flow rate to see whether it is adequate, and therefore normal. All it requires is a measuring cup and a watch with a second hand: With a full bladder, begin urinating. When the stream becomes full, urinate into the cup for ten seconds, then move the cup away. Normal urine flow is 20 cubic centimeters per second (the range is 15–25 cc), so if your cup holds 200 cc (7 or 8 ounces) after ten seconds, you're right on the mark. If it holds noticeably less, see your doctor. If it holds more, that's fine. Another simple test is to write your initials in the snow.

CHAPTER THIRTEEN

Sex Hints

Play a Little. Don't be short on foreplay. Being too eager to get to intercourse is probably the number-one problem of most men. Men who take their time get the results.

Talk About It. Tell your mate what you like and ask what he or she likes best. Don't worry so much about whether you or your partner will have an orgasm. The big O will happen when it happens.

Enjoy Yourself. Sex should be fun, not a race or a performance goal.

Slow Down. You miss a lot of scenery when you drive too fast down a country road. Set the stage yourself: devote more time to sex play.

Take Turns. A lot of men complain that women are too passive. They could help by trading off and encouraging the woman to take turns being the aggressor.

Bathe. Even if you have a long-term mate, don't neglect personal hygiene. A shower or bath before sex will make it nicer for you both.

Don't Worry About Size. Men worry about penis size more than women do. You might be surprised to find that a compact model will do as well as a larger version. And if you have a larger version, be careful and considerate with your partner.

Check All Body Parts. Pay loving attention to other parts of your partner's body—feet, legs, hands, back—as well as the usual erotic areas.

Learn to Laugh. The ability to laugh at yourself or the situation is very important. Laughter defuses tension, especially in a state of failure.

Praise. Make your partner feel special and she or he will make you feel special.

Take a Vacation. Rest and relaxation help, this time and the next time.

Talk and Touch. These are more important than intercourse. Share feelings—it is like dating.

Keep Healthy. Exercise and diet are important in keeping your body in condition. The American Cancer Society recommends common sense and nutrition as guides to good health. Research is under way to evaluate and clarify the role of diet in the development of cancer. So far, no direct cause-and-effect relationship has been proven, but we do know that some things you eat may increase or decrease your risks for certain types of cancer. Based on evidence at hand, you may lessen your chances for getting cancer by following these simple guidelines:

- Avoid obesity, which is defined as being twenty pounds over the recommended weight for your height and age. (Your physician can give you this information.) Sensible eating habits and regular exercise will help you avoid excessive weight gain.
- Cut down on total fat intake. Eat food that is low in fat to control your body weight more easily.
- Eat more high-fiber foods such as cereals, fresh fruit, and vegetables.
- Include foods rich in vitamins A and C in your daily diet. Choose dark green and deep yellow fresh vegetables and fruit (carrots, spinach, sweet potatoes, peaches, and apricots) as sources of vitamin A. Oranges, grapefruit, strawberries, and green and red peppers are rich in vitamin C.
- Include cruciferous vegetables in your diet. These include cabbage, broccoli, brussels sprouts, kohlrabi, and cauliflower.
- Minimize salt-cured, smoked, and nitrite-cured foods. The American food industry has changed to new processes thought to be less hazardous.
- Drink alcohol only moderately and avoid smoking cigarettes.

CHAPTER FOURTEEN

GLOSSARY OF TERMS

Benign   nonmalignant, noncancerous

Benign prostatic hyperplasia (BPH)   Noncancerous enlargement of the prostate that may cause difficulty in urination because of obstruction

Biopsy   Removal of small sample of tissue, usually by needle, for microscopic examination

Bladder   The body's reservoir for urine

Cancer   Abnormal cell growth that may begin in one organ and spread to nearby organs or other parts of the body; a cancer is also called a malignant tumor

Chemotherapy   Treatment of malignant tumors that uses drugs to kill cancer cells

Constriction device   Mechanical device used to contain the blood in the penis in order to sustain an erection; sometimes used with a vacuum device that engorges the penis with blood

Digital rectal examination   Insertion of a gloved, lubricated finger into the rectum to feel the prostate gland

Ejaculation   Release of semen from the penis during orgasm or climax

Epididymis   An elongated pouch on the back of the testicle where sperm mature

Glans penis   The head of the penis

Hormonal therapy   Use of medications or surgical removal of the testicles to prevent male hormones from stimulating further growth of prostate cancer

Impotence   Inability to get an erection and maintain it through intercourse

Injection therapy   The use of a syringe and needle to inject a drug into the penis for the purpose of obtaining an erection

Irradiation therapy   X-ray or other radiation treatment for cancer

Lymph nodes   Small glands located in many areas of the body, including the groin and armpits, that produce substances that help defend the body against invading foreign particles.

Malignant   Cancerous

Metastasis   Spread of cancer to other, sometimes distant, organs

Penile prosthesis   An artificial substitute for a penile erection

Penis   The male sexual organ, six inches long, more or less, when erect

Perineum   The space between the anus and back of the scrotum, about where a bicycle seat hits your bottom

Prostate acid phosphatase (PAP)   Measurement of a substance in the blood produced by prostate cells; the count is elevated in prostate-cancer patients when cancer has spread beyond the prostate.

Prostate (not *prostrate*) gland   A male organ that surrounds the neck of the bladder and the urethra and produces some seminal fluid

Prostate specific antigen (PSA) test   Measurement of the level in the blood of a certain protein produced by both benign and malignant prostate cells

Prostatectomy   Surgical removal of the entire prostate gland (radical prostatectomy) or a portion of it (transurethral resection) (*see* TURP)

Prostatitis   Inflammation of the prostate gland

Scrotum   The sack that holds and covers the testicles

Semen (seminal fluid, ejaculate)   A thick, whitish secretion from male reproductive organs

Seminal vesicles   Paired pouches behind the prostate that produce most of a man's seminal fluid

Testicles   Male gonads that produce sperm and hormones; also called testes

Testosterone   A male sex hormone produced in the testicles

Transrectal ultrasonography   An ultrasound examination of the prostate in which a probe inserted into the rectum uses sound waves to produce an image of the prostate on a television screen.

TURP (transurethral resection of the prostate)   A surgical operation that removes growths within the prostate but spares the gland, comparable to removing pulp in an orange but leaving the rind.

Urethral   The tube that runs from the bladder through the penis to convey urine and seminal fluid

Urethritis   An inflammation of the urethra

Urologist An investigator of a man's private parts

Vas deferens Tubes that carry sperm from the epididymis to ejaculatory ducts in the prostate

Vasectomy An operation that severs the vas deferens to render a man sterile

CHAPTER FIFTEEN

INTERNET REFERENCES

It's time to take control of your own health and know more about your own body. Women are much more acquainted with their health and health issues than men are, and men have a lot of catching up to do. Men's fear of the unknown is the reason, the big reason why people, especially men, do not want to see their doctor. They are afraid of what they will find; therefore, they avoid the doctor at all costs. Women frequently will encourage their husbands and loved ones to go to the doctor to see what is going on, a habit they have probably developed through experience with PAP smears and mammograms over the years. So, men, get your heads out of the sand and get to know your body—and live longer. Knowledge and lifestyle changes can extend your life in a healthy way.

The amount of health-care information available on the Internet increases daily and should be utilized by patients and doctors alike to learn and to help devise the most up-to-date care for patients' particular situations. The benefit of using the Internet is that it is for the most part strictly confidential and can be done on your own time. Listed here, then, are a number of Internet sites and Web pages I recommend for men and women interested in investigating men's private parts. Most of them are updated regularly, with the latest update is usually included in special segments.

PROSTATE

http://cancernet.nci.nih.gov/Cancer_Types/Prostate_Cancer.shtml
http://www.prostate.com/
http://www.aoa.dhhs.gov/aoa/pages/agepages/prostate.html

BLADDER

http://cancernet.nci.nih.gov/cancer_types/bladder_cancer.shtml

TESTICLE

http://cancernet.nci.nih.gov/cancer_Types/Testicular_cancer.shtml

UROLOGY

http://www.afud.org/home.html or 800-242-2383
http://www.auanet.org/index_hi.cfm
http://www.noah.cuny.cdu/

References

Barry, M. J., et al. "The American Association Symptom Index for Benign Prostatic Hyperplasia." *Journal of Urology* 148 (1992):1549–57.

Gilbaugh, J., and P. Fuchs. *The Gonococcus and the Toilet Seat. New England Journal of Medicine* 301 (July 12, 1979): 91–93.

McConnell, J. D., et al. *Benign Prostatic Hyperplasia: Diagnosis and Treatment.* Clinical practice guideline no. 8, Agency for Health Care Policy and Research publication no. 94-0582. Rockville, Md.: Agency for Health Care Policy and Research, Public Health Service, U.S. Department of Health and Human Services, February 1994.

Oesterling, J. E., et al. Influence of Patient Age on the Serum PSA Concentration. *Urological Clinicians of North America* 20 (1993):671.

INDEX